Nano-Micro Encapsulation of Drugs

Nano-Micro Encapsulation of Drugs

Editors

Beatriz Clares
Ana C. Calpena

MDPI • Basel • Beijing • Wuhan • Barcelona • Belgrade • Manchester • Tokyo • Cluj • Tianjin

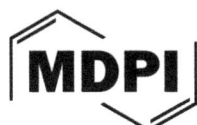

Editors
Beatriz Clares
Pharmacy and Pharmaceutical
Technology
University of Granada
Granada
Spain

Ana C. Calpena
Pharmacy, Pharmaceutical
Technology and
Physical-Chemistry
University of Barcelona
Barcelona
Spain

Editorial Office
MDPI
St. Alban-Anlage 66
4052 Basel, Switzerland

This is a reprint of articles from the Special Issue published online in the open access journal *Pharmaceutics* (ISSN 1999-4923) (available at: www.mdpi.com/journal/pharmaceutics/special_issues/encapsulation2020).

For citation purposes, cite each article independently as indicated on the article page online and as indicated below:

LastName, A.A.; LastName, B.B.; LastName, C.C. Article Title. *Journal Name* **Year**, *Volume Number*, Page Range.

ISBN 978-3-0365-2945-5 (Hbk)
ISBN 978-3-0365-2944-8 (PDF)

© 2022 by the authors. Articles in this book are Open Access and distributed under the Creative Commons Attribution (CC BY) license, which allows users to download, copy and build upon published articles, as long as the author and publisher are properly credited, which ensures maximum dissemination and a wider impact of our publications.

The book as a whole is distributed by MDPI under the terms and conditions of the Creative Commons license CC BY-NC-ND.

Contents

About the Editors vii

Preface to "Nano-Micro Encapsulation of Drugs" ix

Eliana B. Souto, Selma B. Souto, Aleksandra Zielinska, Alessandra Durazzo, Massimo Lucarini, Antonello Santini, Olaf K. Horbańczuk, Atanas G. Atanasov, Conrado Marques, Luciana N. Andrade, Amélia M. Silva and Patricia Severino
Perillaldehyde 1,2-epoxide Loaded SLN-Tailored mAb: Production, Physicochemical Characterization and In Vitro Cytotoxicity Profile in MCF-7 Cell Lines
Reprinted from: *Pharmaceutics* **2020**, *12*, 161, doi:10.3390/pharmaceutics12020161 1

Suhair Sunoqrot, Malek Alfaraj, Ala'a M. Hammad, Violet Kasabri, Dana Shalabi, Ahmad A. Deeb, Lina Hasan Ibrahim, Khaldoun Shnewer and Ismail Yousef
Development of a Thymoquinone Polymeric Anticancer Nanomedicine through Optimization of Polymer Molecular Weight and Nanoparticle Architecture
Reprinted from: *Pharmaceutics* **2020**, *12*, 811, doi:10.3390/pharmaceutics12090811 15

Sandra Giraldo, María E. Alea-Reyes, David Limón, Asensio González, Marta Duch, José A. Plaza, David Ramos-López, Joaquín de Lapuente, Arántzazu González-Campo and Lluïsa Pérez-García
π-Donor/π-Acceptor Interactions for the Encapsulation of Neurotransmitters on Functionalized Polysilicon-Based Microparticles
Reprinted from: *Pharmaceutics* **2020**, *12*, 724, doi:10.3390/pharmaceutics12080724 31

Nemany A. N. Hanafy, Isabel Fabregat, Stefano Leporatti and Maged El Kemary
Encapsulating TGF-β1 Inhibitory Peptides P17 and P144 as a Promising Strategy to Facilitate Their Dissolution and to Improve Their Functionalization
Reprinted from: *Pharmaceutics* **2020**, *12*, 421, doi:10.3390/pharmaceutics12050421 51

Maria Aurora Grimaudo, Angel Concheiro and Carmen Alvarez-Lorenzo
Crosslinked Hyaluronan Electrospun Nanofibers for Ferulic Acid Ocular Delivery
Reprinted from: *Pharmaceutics* **2020**, *12*, 274, doi:10.3390/pharmaceutics12030274 69

Paola Mura, Francesca Maestrelli, Mario D'Ambrosio, Cristina Luceri and Marzia Cirri
Evaluation and Comparison of Solid Lipid Nanoparticles (SLNs) and Nanostructured Lipid Carriers (NLCs) as Vectors to Develop Hydrochlorothiazide Effective and Safe Pediatric Oral Liquid Formulations
Reprinted from: *Pharmaceutics* **2021**, *13*, 437, doi:10.3390/pharmaceutics13040437 83

Eloy Pena-Rodríguez, Mari Carmen Moreno, Bárbara Blanco-Fernandez, Jordi González and Francisco Fernández-Campos
Epidermal Delivery of Retinyl Palmitate Loaded Transfersomes: Penetration and Biodistribution Studies
Reprinted from: *Pharmaceutics* **2020**, *12*, 112, doi:10.3390/pharmaceutics12020112 101

José L. Soriano, Ana C. Calpena, María J. Rodríguez-Lagunas, Òscar Domènech, Nuria Bozal-de Febrer, María L. Garduño-Ramírez and Beatriz Clares
Endogenous Antioxidant Cocktail Loaded Hydrogel for Topical Wound Healing of Burns
Reprinted from: *Pharmaceutics* **2020**, *13*, 8, doi:10.3390/pharmaceutics13010008 115

About the Editors

Prof. Beatriz Clares is affiliated with the Department of Pharmacy and Pharmaceutical Technology, University of Granada, Spain. She graduated in Pharmaceutical Sciences from the same University (1997), achieving her Ph.D. in Pharmaceutical Technology at the University of Granada (2003). She joined the University of Granada as an Assistant Professor in 2007, obtaining a permanent post in 2013. She is a member of the Institute of Nanoscience and Nanotechnology of the University of Barcelona, Biosanitary Research Institute of Granada, Controlled Release Society, Spanish Society of Pharmacology, and Technological Institute of Individualized Medicines. Her research focuses on the design, development, and characterization of new drug delivery systems, including the controlled delivery of drugs across biological barriers, with special emphasis for skin and mucosa administration. She has wide experience in publishing scientific research. She also acts as a reviewer in various international journals. Due to her merits, in 2019 she was awarded the -American Academy of Pharmacy Award, for her work throughout her scientific career.

Prof. Ana Cristina Calpena is a full professor at the Department of Pharmacy and Pharmaceutical Technology and Physical Chemistry at the Faculty of Pharmacy and Food Sciences, University of Barcelona, Spain. She leads the research group NanoBioPharma in the Institute of Nanoscience and Nanotechnology of the University of Barcelona (IN2UB). Her research experience encompasses the biopharmaceutical and pharmacokinetic study of all types of drugs and active ingredients, particularly through skin, as well as ocular, oral, and vaginal mucosa. She is currently focused on the field of nanobiomedicine, including the use of nano/microparticulate liquid and semi-solid formulations for drug delivery. Due to her research carried out previous years, she participates as a researcher in various projects and financed contracts in the pharmaceutical industry, whose resulting products are marketed in different countries.

Preface to "Nano-Micro Encapsulation of Drugs"

The encapsulation of drugs in nano/micro-vehicles is a tremendously challenging task which is continuously evolving. The development of nano/micro-carriers is among the most important areas of pharmaceutical and biomedical research. This process provides several possibilities to facilitate drug protection and delivery at specific biological sites, among many other benefits. These two techniques (nano- and microencapsulation), as well as other relevant aspects related to optimization, cover a wide range of drug carriers, from nanoparticles, nanospheres, nanocapsules, etc., to their microsized counterparts, as well as other colloidal drug delivery systems such as liposomes, micelles, nanoemulsions, and microemulsions, among others. Thus, different materials, methods of production, possibilities of surface modification, and targetability options need to be considered. Further research into this field would certainly help to improve the therapeutic tools available at present. For this reason, this Special Issue is aimed at a wide audience of people related to the fields of nanotechnology, material science, medicine, etc.

This Special Issue also covers different aspects of the nano/microencapsulation of drugs, including papers describing the design, preparation, and characterization of nano- and micro-carrier-based drug delivery systems and the latest developments in key fields. Eight articles regarding this topic were selected for this Special Issue, demonstrating the potential of this development strategy for drug delivery in a wide range of applications (from cancer treatment to wound healing, as well as cardiovascular or ocular diseases). Prestigious experts in these fields have participated in this Special Issue, sharing their research and contributions with authors affiliated with different Universities and other renowned and well-respected institutions.

The guest editors wish to express their gratitude to all authors and collaborators that have contributed to this Special Issue, as well as the Assistant Editors of *Pharmaceutics*.

Beatriz Clares, Ana C. Calpena
Editors

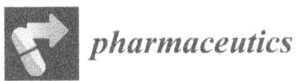 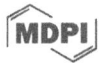

Article

Perillaldehyde 1,2-epoxide Loaded SLN-Tailored mAb: Production, Physicochemical Characterization and In Vitro Cytotoxicity Profile in MCF-7 Cell Lines

Eliana B. Souto [1,2,*], Selma B. Souto [3], Aleksandra Zielinska [1], Alessandra Durazzo [4], Massimo Lucarini [4], Antonello Santini [5,*], Olaf K. Horbańczuk [6], Atanas G. Atanasov [7,8,9,10], Conrado Marques [11,12,13], Luciana N. Andrade [14,15], Amélia M. Silva [16,17] and Patricia Severino [11,12,13,*]

[1] Department of Pharmaceutical Technology, Faculty of Pharmacy (FFUC), University of Coimbra, Pólo das Ciências da Saúde, Azinhaga de Santa Comba, 3000-548 Coimbra, Portugal; zielinska-aleksandra@wp.pl
[2] CEB—Centre of Biological Engineering, University of Minho, Campus de Gualtar 4710-057 Braga, Portugal
[3] Department of Endocrinology, Hospital de São João, Alameda Prof. Hernâni Monteiro, 4200-319 Porto, Portugal; sbsouto.md@gmail.com
[4] CREA-Research Centre for Food and Nutrition, Via Ardeatina 546, 00178 Rome, Italy; alessandra.durazzo@crea.gov.it (A.D.); massimo.lucarini@crea.gov.it (M.L.)
[5] Department of Pharmacy, University of Napoli Federico II, 80131 Napoli, Italy
[6] Department of Technique and Food Product Development, Warsaw University of Life Sciences (WULS-SGGW) 159c Nowoursynowska, 02-776 Warsaw, Poland; olaf_horbanczuk@sggw.pl
[7] Institute of Neurobiology, Bulgarian Academy of Sciences, 23 Acad. G. Bonchev str., 1113 Sofia, Bulgaria; atanas.atanasov@univie.ac.at
[8] Institute of Genetics and Animal Breeding, Polish Academy of Sciences, Jastrzębiec, 05-552 Magdalenka, Poland
[9] Department of Pharmacognosy, University of Vienna, Althanstraße 14, 1090 Vienna, Austria
[10] Ludwig Boltzmann Institute for Digital Health and Patient Safety, Medical University of Vienna, Spitalgasse 23, 1090 Vienna, Austria
[11] Laboratory of Nanotechnology and Nanomedicine (LNMED), Institute of Technology and Research (ITP), Av. Murilo Dantas 300, Aracaju 49010-390, Brazil; conrado.marques@souunit.com.br
[12] Industrial Biotechnology Program, University of Tiradentes (UNIT); Av. Murilo Dantas 300, Aracaju 49032-490, Brazil
[13] Tiradentes Institute, 150 Mt Vernon St, Dorchester, MA 02125, USA
[14] Laboratory of Nanotechnology and Nanomedicine, Institute of Technology and Research, Aracaju SE 49032-490, Brazil; luciana.nalone@hotmail.com
[15] School of Pharmacy, University Tiradentes, Aracaju SE 49032-490, Brazil
[16] School of Biology and Environment, University of Trás-os-Montes e Alto Douro (UTAD), Quinta de Prados, P-5001-801 Vila Real, Portugal; amsilva@utad.pt
[17] Centre for Research and Technology of Agro-Environmental and Biological Sciences (CITAB), University of Trás-os-Montes e Alto Douro (UTAD), P-5001-801 Vila Real, Portugal
* Correspondence: ebsouto@ff.uc.pt (E.B.S.); asantini@unina.it (A.S.); patricia_severino@itp.org.br (P.S.); Tel.: +351-239-488-400 (E.B.S.); Tel.: +39-81-253-9317 (A.S.); +55-79-3218-2190 (P.S.)

Received: 20 January 2020; Accepted: 13 February 2020; Published: 16 February 2020

Abstract: We have developed a new cationic solid lipid nanoparticle (SLN) formulation, composed of Compritol ATO 888, poloxamer 188 and cetyltrimethylammonium bromide (CTAB), to load perillaldehyde 1,2-epoxide, and surface-tailored with a monoclonal antibody for site-specific targeting of human epithelial growth receptor 2 (HER2). Perillaldehyde 1,2-epoxide-loaded cationic SLN (cPa-SLN), with a mean particle size (z-Ave) of 275.31 ± 4.78 nm and polydispersity index (PI) of 0.303 ± 0.081, were produced by high shear homogenization. An encapsulation efficiency of cPa-SLN above 80% was achieved. The release of perillaldehyde 1,2-epoxide from cationic SLN followed the Korsemeyer–Peppas kinetic model, which is typically seen in nanoparticle formulations. The lipid peroxidation of cPa-SLN was assessed by the capacity to produce thiobarbituric acid-reactive substances, while the antioxidant activity was determined by the capacity to scavenge the stable radical DPPH. The surface functionalization of c*Pa*-SLN with the antibody was done via streptavidin-biotin interaction, monitoring z-Ave, PI and ZP of the obtained assembly (c*Pa*-SLN-S_{Ab}), as well as its stability in phosphate buffer. The effect of plain cationic SLN (c-SLN, monoterpene free), c*Pa*-SLN and c*Pa*-SLN-S_{Ab} onto the MCF-7 cell lines was evaluated in a concentration range from 0.01 to 0.1 mg/mL, confirming that streptavidin adsorption onto c*Pa*-SLN-S_{Ab} improved the cell viability in comparison to the cationic c*Pa*-SLN.

Keywords: perillaldehyde 1,2-epoxide; Compritol ATO 888; cationic SLN; streptavidin adsorption; MCF-7 cells

1. Introduction

The nonselective delivery of anticancer drugs to the tumor site remains a challenge in chemotherapy and is the reason for the serious side effects of the classical treatments. Nanoparticles have partially solved this limitation, by reducing the systemic distribution of anticancer drugs by passive targeting. Cationic nanoparticles with a net positive surface charge have been proposed to further enhance cellular interaction and increase the cellular uptake of the loaded drug [1–6]. Site-specific delivery can be achieved via active targeting by surface modifying, such as with antibodies, aptamers and other targeting moieties (e.g., transferrin, folate) tailored to specific receptors [7,8].

Traditional medicine has countless of examples of natural compounds with several health benefits. Essential oils are indeed a source of phytochemicals of pharmaceutical and nutraceutical interest, with monoterpenes being their main constituents [9]. Monoterpenes show antioxidant, antimicrobial, analgesic, anxiolytic and anticancer properties, with an increasing interest as a source of therapeutic alternatives [10–13]. Perillyl alcohol, a naturally occurring monoterpene found in the essential oils peppermint and lavender, has been widely studied [14], demonstrating effectiveness against a variety of human tumor cell lines [15–17]. The monoterpene showed cytotoxicity and antitumor activity in various experimental models, and has already reached clinical trials for cancer treatment [15,18]. The cytotoxicity of perillyl alcohol analogues, such as (-)-8,9-perillaldehyde epoxide, (-)-perillaldehyde, (+)-limonene 1,2-epoxide and (-)-8-hydroxycarvotanacetone, has also been thoroughly characterized [15]. The anti-tumoral activity of perillaldehyde 1,2-epoxide has also been described by Andrade et al. [15,19]. The aim of this study has been the loading of perillaldehyde 1,2-epoxide into cationic solid lipid nanoparticles (cSLN) for site-specific delivery to breast cancer cells. Solid lipid nanoparticles (SLN) have been selected as a delivery system due to their composition in biocompatible and biodegradable lipids, with a reduced risk of cyto/genotoxic events [3,20,21]. Furthermore, these particles can be produced with cationic lipids so that the positive charge can then be functionalized with a monoclonal antibody against human epithelial growth receptor 2 (HER2) [8].

2. Materials and Methods

2.1. Materials

Compritol ATO 888 (glycerol behenate) was obtained as a gift from Gattefosse (Saint-Priest, France), Poloxamer 188 (trade name: Kolliphor® P188) was bought from BASF (Ludwigshafen, Germany), the ErbB2/HER-2 monoclonal antibody (CB11) was obtained from ThermoFisher Scientific (Wilmington, USA) and cetyltrimethylammonium bromide (CTAB) was purchased from Sigma (Sintra, Portugal). Perillaldehyde, 3-(4,5-dimethyl-2-thiazolyl)-2,5-diphenyl-2H-tetrazolium bromide (MTT), doxorubicin (purity > 98%), Trolox, thiobarbituric acid (TBA), butylated hydroxytoluene (BHT), dimethyl sulfoxide (DMSO), methanol, hexane, ethyl acetate, hydrogen peroxide (30%) and potassium hydroxide were purchased from Sigma Chemical Co. (St. Louis, MO, USA). Double-distilled water was used throughout the work, after filtration in a MiliQ system (Millipore, Merck KGaA, Darmstadt, Germany).

2.2. Synthesis of Perillaldehyde 1,2-epoxide

The synthesis of perillaldehyde 1,2-epoxide was carried out as described by Andrade et al. [19], who analyzed the product by infrared and ^{1}H- and ^{13}C-NMR [15]. Briefly, a solution of 7.5% (m/v) perillaldehyde in methanol was mixed with hydrogen peroxide (30%) in a 250 mL flask, and kept in an ice bath (0–4 °C), to which a volume of 5 mL of potassium hydroxide (0.5 g/mL) was added dropwise. The reaction medium was stirred for a period of four hours, after which it was removed from the ice bath and the aqueous phase was extracted by washing it with 50 mL of dichloromethane. The organic phase was washed twice with 50 mL double-distilled water, dried with anhydrous sodium sulfate and concentrated in an IKA rotary evaporator (Staufen, Germany). Purification was done in a silica gel column chromatography, using a mixture of hexane/ethyl acetate (9:1) as eluant. A yield of 77.8% was obtained for perillaldehyde 1,2-epoxide.

2.3. Production of Cationic Solid Lipid Nanoparticles (cSLN)

2.3.1. Non-Functionalized cSLN

The production of cationic SLN (cSLN) was carried out by hot high-shear homogenization, as described by Souto et al. [8], using glycerol behenate as solid lipid and poloxamer 188 as surfactant. Compritol (glycerol behenate) [5.0% (w/v)] was melted at 80 °C and then dispersed in an aqueous solution composed of 0.25% (w/v) poloxamer 188 and 0.5% (w/v) CTAB, heated up at the same temperature to produce an emulsion under stirring at 8000 rpm for 10 min in an Ultra-Turrax (Ultra-Turrax ®, T25, IKA, Staufen, Germany). The obtained emulsion was diluted (2:1) in cold water, kept at 4 ± 0.5 °C and further processed at 5000 rpm for five more minutes. The obtained particles were transferred to siliconized glass vials and stored at 4 ± 0.5 °C for further studies. For the loading of cSLN with the synthesized perillaldehyde 1,2-epoxide (cPa-SLN), nanoparticles were produced as described, by adding the drug [0.5% (w/w)] to the melted lipid [4.5% (w/v)] prior to emulsification. Weightings were done in an analytical balance (Mettler Toledo, Giessen, Germany) with a readability of 0.005 mg.

2.3.2. mAb-Functionalized cSLN

The functionalization of cPa-SLN was carried out as previously described, and following the method proposed by Petersen et al. [22]. Firstly, the ability of the produced cationic nanoparticles to bind streptavidin was evaluated by incubating cPa-SLN with the protein at decreasing ratios (1:5, 1:10, 1:15, 1:20 and 1:25), for a period of one hour at room temperature. The formation of the cPa-SLN-Streptavidin (cPa-SLN-S) complexes was monitored by determining z-AVE and ZP, as described in 2.4. The monoclonal antibody (mAb, CB11) was dispersed in PBS (pH 7.4), diluted down to 1 mg/mL and biotinylated using a Biotinylation Kit (Biotin Conjugation Kit (Fast, Type A) Lightning-Link®). Aliquots of biotinylated antibody were stored at −20 °C until further use. cPa-SLN-S complexes were mixed with a biotinylated antibody and incubated at room temperature over at least one hour to complex with the mAb, and form cPa-SLN-S_{Ab} complexes. The formation of the cPa-SLN-S_{Ab} complexes (i.e., the adsorption of mAb onto the cPa-SLN-S surface) was monitored by measuring z-AVE and ZP, as described in Section 2.4.

2.4. Mean Particle Size, Polydispersity Index and Zeta Potential

Immediately after the production of each nanoparticle batch, the mean particle size (z-Ave) and polydispersity index (PI) were determined by dynamic light scattering (DLS, Zetasizer Nano ZS, Malvern, Worcestershire, UK). Prior to the analysis of cSLN and cPa-SLN, particles were diluted with MilliQ water and measured at a 1 mg/mL of solid lipid concentration. Prior to the analysis of cPa-SLN-S and cPa-SLN-S_{Ab}, particles were diluted in a phosphate buffer saline (PBS, pH 7.4) and measured at a 1 mg/mL of solid lipid concentration. Zeta potential (ZP) was recorded in a laser Doppler anemometry Zetasizer Nano ZS (Malvern, Worcestershire, UK) using the Smoluchowski equation. Dilutions were performed prior to analysis, as described for the recording of z-Ave and PI. Measurements were done in triplicate (n = 3) (10 runs per measurement, 30 in total), and data were expressed as the arithmetical mean ± standard deviation (SD).

2.5. Encapsulation Efficiency (EE)

The encapsulation efficiency (EE) of perillaldehyde 1,2-epoxide in cPa-SLN was determined as an indirect measure of the amount of drug quantified in supernatant [23]. Briefly, cPa-SLN was firstly ultra-centrifuged for 1 h at 100,000 g in a Beckman Optima™ Ultracentrifuge (Optima™ XL, Indianapolis, IN, USA) and the quantification of perillaldehyde 1,2-epoxide, determined in the supernatant in a UV spectrophotometer Shimadzu UV-1601 (Shimadzu Italy, Cornaredo, Italy), at 245 nm. The following equation was used to calculate EE% [24]

$$EE\% = \frac{W_{Pa} - W_s}{W_{Pa}} \times 100 \qquad (1)$$

where W_{PA} is the mass of perillaldehyde 1,2-epoxide used for the production of SLN, and W_S is the mass of perillaldehyde 1,2-epoxide quantified in the supernatant.

2.6. In Vitro Release Profile of cPa-SLN

Vertical Franz diffusion cells were used to determine the in vitro release profile of perillaldehyde 1,2-epoxide from cPa-SLN. Prior to the assay, cellulose membranes with an average pore size of 0.22 μm (MERCK KgaA, Darmstadt, Germany) were firstly soaked for 2 h in PBS (pH 7.4), and then placed between the donor and acceptor compartments. A volume of 1 mL of freshly prepared cPa-SLN was placed onto the top of the donor compartment. The acceptor compartment, containing 5 mL of a PBS buffer, was kept under magnetic stirring at 37 °C over the course of the assay. At pre-determined time intervals, a volume of 200 μL was sampled with a syringe, being the same volume replaced with the PBS buffer to ensure sink conditions. The cumulative amount of perillaldehyde 1,2-epoxide was analysed in a UV spectrophotometer Shimadzu UV-1601 (Shimadzu Italy, Cornaredo, Italy) at 245 nm. Four kinetic models, namely the zero order, first order, Higuchi and Korsmeyer-Peppas models, have been used for the mathematical fitting of the recorded values [25]. The obtained R^2 values were used for the selection of the most appropriate model.

2.7. In Vitro Lipid Peroxidation Assay

To 1 mL of egg yolk homogenate (1% w/v) in phosphate buffer (pH 7.4), a volume of 0.1 mL ferrous sulphate ($FeSO_4$, 0.17 mol/L) was added. To the obtained mixture, increasing concentrations of cPa-SLN (1, 2, 3, 4, 5 and 10 μg/mL, solid lipid) were added, which were then incubated at 37 °C for 30 min. After cooling, a volume of 0.5 mL of each mixture was centrifuged with 0.5 mL of trichloroacetic acid solution (15% m/v) for 10 min at 1200 rpm. The collected supernatant (0.5 mL) was mixed with the same volume of thiobarbituric acid solution (0.67% m/v) and incubated for 60 min at 95 °C. After cooling, the formation of TBARS was quantified by spectrophotometry by measuring the supernatant at 532 nm, and the results were expressed as malondialdehyde equivalents (MDA Eq) of the substrate. Trolox (standard antioxidant) was used as positive control, at 50 μg/mL, against water as the negative control.

2.8. In Vitro Antioxidant Activity of cPa-SLN

The antioxidant activity of cPa-SLN was determined as the ability of the loaded drug to scavenge the stable radical DPPH• [26]. Briefly, cPa-SLN was firstly dissolved in 0.1 mM of a DPPH methanolic solution to achieve concentrations of cPa-SLN of 1, 2, 3, 4, 5 and 10 μg/mL of solid lipid. Then, 20 μL of samples were placed in the microplate wells. Finally, 200 μL DPPH methanolic solution (0.1 mM), were added to each of the wells. Methanol and butylated hydroxytoluene (BHT, 0–6 μg/mL) were used as negative and positive controls, respectively. The microplates were incubated at 25 °C for 30 min, and then read at 517 nm in a multiplate reader (DTX 880 Multimode Detector, Beckman Coulter Inc.). The antioxidant activity (AA) as the measure of the percentage of scavenging of free radicals was calculated from the recorded optical densities (OD), using the following equation:

$$AA\% = \frac{\text{OD of negative control} - \text{OD of sample}}{\text{OD of negative control}} \times 100 \quad (2)$$

By plotting the concentration in the X-axis (μg/mL) against $AA\%$ in the Y-axis (% inhibition), the linear regression equation was obtained and the IC_{50} value determined.

2.9. Cell Culture and MTT Assay

The cytotoxicity of cSLN (blank) and c*Pa*-SLN was tested in MCF-7 cells obtained from ATCC (Pensabio Biotecnologia, São Paulo, Brazil). Cells were cultured in RPMI-1640 medium supplemented with 10% fetal bovine serum, 2 mM L-glutamine, 100 μg/mL streptomycin and 100 U/mL penicillin, and further incubated at 37 °C in a 5% CO_2 atmosphere. Consumables for cell culture were obtained from Sigma Chemical Co. (St. Louis, MO, USA). For the 3-(4,5-dimethyl-2-thiazolyl)-2,5-diphenyl-2H-tetrazolium bromide (MTT) assay [27], cells were incubated in 96-well plates (0.1 × 10^6 cells/mL; 100 μL/well) for 24 h. Solutions of cSLN (blank) and c*Pa*-SLN in dimethyl sulfoxide (DMSO 0.7%) at increasing concentrations (1, 2, 3, 4, 5 and 10 μg/mL of solid lipid) were added to each well, and incubated for more 72 h at 37 °C in a 5% CO_2 atmosphere. A solution of DMSO 1% was set as the negative control, whereas a doxorubicin solution (100 μg/mL) was set as the positive control. At the end of the incubation period, test solutions were removed. An MTT solution (150 μL) at 0.5 mg/mL was added to each well, and incubated for three hours at 37 °C in a 5% CO_2 atmosphere. Cell viability was determined as the ability of viable cells to reduce the yellow dye MTT to the purple formazan. The obtained precipitate was dissolved in 150 μL DMSO, and the absorbance was read at 595 nm using a multiplate reader (DTX 880 Multimode Detector, Beckman Coulter Inc.). The results were expressed as percentage of cell growth inhibition (%GI) as follows:

$$\%GI = 100 \times \left[\frac{Abs_{Test}}{Abs_{Negative\ Control}} \times 100 \right] \quad (3)$$

2.10. Statistical Analysis

Data obtained are expressed as the mean ± SEM, and the differences among experimental groups were evaluated using a one-way analysis of variance (ANOVA) followed by the Dunnet post-test. Values of $p < 0.05$ were considered significant. All statistical analyses were carried using the GraphPad program 5.0® (Intuitive Software for Science, San Diego, CA, USA).

3. Results and Discussion

From the *p*-menthane derivatives described by Andrade et al. [15], perillaldehyde 1,2-epoxide was selected due to its high cytotoxic profile (growth inhibition ($GI\%$) > 95%), and was tested in a concentration of 25 μg/mL in colon carcinoma (HCT-116), ovarian adenocarcinoma (OVCAR-8), glioblastoma (SF-295) and promyelocytic leucemia (HL-60) cell lines [19]. Literature states that $GI\%$ = 0 means no cytotoxicity, while 1 < $GI\%$ < 50 is low cytotoxicity, 51 < $GI\%$ < 75 is moderate cytotoxicity and $GI\%$ > 75 is cytotoxicity [28]. To reduce the cytotoxicity of the compound while increasing site-specific delivery, we proposed the loading of perillaldehyde 1,2-epoxide into cationic solid lipid nanoparticles (SLN), to be surface tailored to HER2 receptors. The loading of the selected monoterpene into Compritol cSLN resulted in particles with the characteristics summarized in Table 1. The high-shear homogenization method has been previously shown to produce SLN of a low mean size and polydispersity [8], and the possibility to operate at a temperature compatible with the thermal stability of the selected drug [15,29].

Table 1. Mean particle size (z-AVE), polydispersity index (PI), zeta potential (ZP) and encapsulation efficiency (EE%) of perillaldehyde 1,2-epoxide into cationic SLN.

Batch	z-Ave (nm)	PI	ZP (mV)	EE%
cSLN	217.89 ± 5.33	0.293 ± 0.049	+67.91 ± 3.41	–
cPa-SLN	275.31 ± 4.76	0.303 ± 0.081	+65.57 ± 2.23	81.64 ± 1.06

The nonsurface modified cationic SLN showed a very high positive net charge in both batches, due to the presence of CTAB (0.5% m/v) on the surface. Both z-Ave and PI increased with the loading of the monoterpene, showing a slightly broad distribution with a PI above 0.24 (values below this limit are considered monodispersed). A slight decrease of ZP was found with the loading of perillaldehyde 1,2-epoxide, attributed to its lipophilic character, and confirming its loading within the lipid matrices.

Due to its lipophilic character, more than 80% of the drug was encapsulated within Compritol matrices. As SLN are of a crystalline nature, it is expected that a modified release profile can be achieved for the loaded drug. The release profile of cPa-SLN was evaluated over the course of 24 h, and the results are shown in Figure 1.

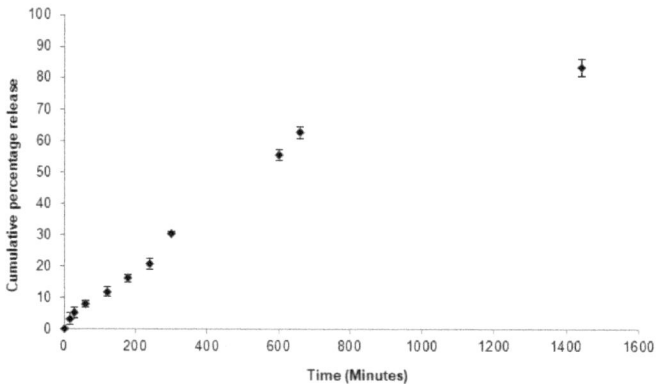

Figure 1. Cumulative percentage release of perillaldehyde 1,2-epoxide from cPa-SLN over 24 h.

About 12% of the drug was released within the first two hours (11.90 ± 1.52%), while at the end of the 24-h period, 83.40 ± 2.79% of the drug was released. The depicted profile cPa-SLN translates a controlled release of perillaldehyde 1,2-epoxide from the cationic particles. To further elucidate which mechanisms are behind such releases, four mathematical models were used to fit the recorded values (Figure 2).

From the values obtained for R^2, the best model describing the release of perillaldehyde 1,2-epoxide from cPa-SLN was shown to be Korsmeyers–Peppas, with a R^2 of 0.9791, the closest straight-line results. This model describes the drug release from the nanoparticles accordingly to $M_t/M_\infty = k't^n$, where M_t is the cumulative amount of the drug released at time t, M_∞ is the cumulative amount of the drug released at an infinite time, k' is the constant that is governed by the physicochemical properties of the nanoparticle matrix and n is the diffusional release exponent indicating of the mechanism of the drug release. Indeed, $n = 0.5$ stands for Fickian diffusion, whereas $0.5 < n < 1.0$ means a non-Fickian diffusion. The shape of the particles plays a significant role on the drug release. For particles of a spherical shape, the drug release becomes independent of time and reaches a zero-order release, known as Case II transport, achieved as n approaches 1.0. In such cases, a diffusional exponent n = 1.0 is indicative of non-Fickian transport. If $n > 1.0$, super Case II transport is followed [30]. The second-best fitting model was Higuchi, with a R^2 of 0.9535. The Higuchi model describes the fraction of the drug released from a matrix being proportional to the square root of time, i.e., $M_t/M_\infty = k_H t^{\frac{1}{2}}$, where M_t is the cumulative amount of the drug released at time t, M_∞ is the cumulative amount of the drug released at an infinite time, and k_H is the Higuchi dissolution constant, which is governed by the physicochemical properties of the nanoparticle matrix. If the release profile follows this model (Fickian diffusion), it means that a straight line with k_H as a slope will be obtained when plotting $x = k_H$ against $y = M_t/M_\infty$. The modified release profile is achieved because of the solid state of the lipid core, as previously confirmed by us [2]. Besides, we have also confirmed by DSC and x-Ray diffraction that cationic surfactant CTAB forms a stabilizing layer on the SLN surface, and is not part of the inner matrix, solely composed of solid lipid and the drug. These results were confirmed by the decrease of ZP over storage time, which means that CTAB may suffer some adsorption from the surface during its shelf life [31].

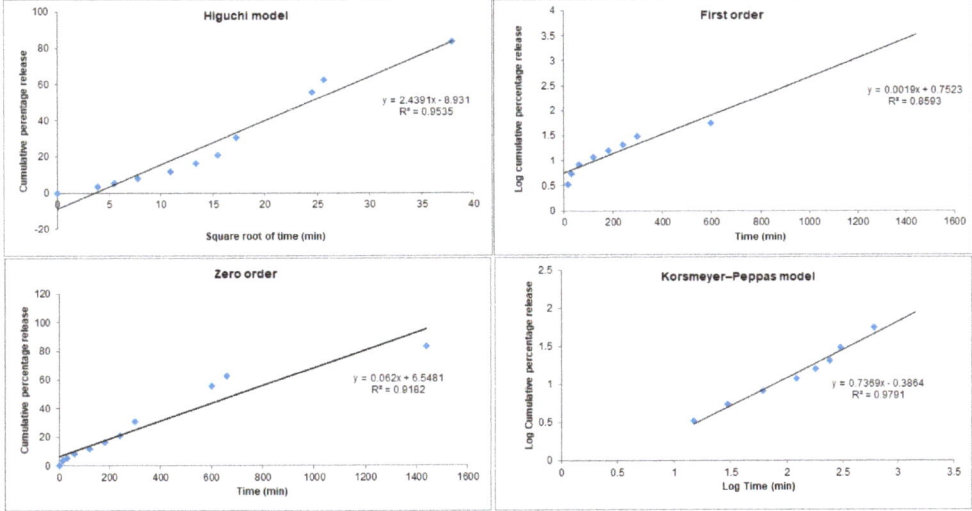

Figure 2. Mathematical fitting models of the release profile of perillaldehyde 1,2-epoxide from cPa-SLN over 24 h.

Due to the vulnerability of lipid materials to free radicals, SLN can suffer lipid peroxidation. However, it is estimated that perillaldehyde 1,2-epoxide, as a monoterpene derivative, can neutralize the free radicals eventually resulting from lipid peroxidation. Increasing concentrations of cPa-SLN (1, 2, 3, 4, 5 and 10 µg/mL) were assayed, and the results are depicted in Figure 3. As shown in Figure 3, the increasing concentration of the particles increased the neutralizing capacity attributed to the higher amount of the drug available to reduce the product formation generated by lipid peroxidation, i.e., the MDA (nmol MDA Eq/mL), when compared to the negative control ($p < 0.05$). The six tested concentrations (1, 2, 3, 4, 5 and 10 µg/mL) revealed an antioxidant effect, i.e., the capacity of cPa-SLN to inhibit the Fenton reaction. This property is also linked to the capacity of terpenes in preventing DNA damage by neutralizing reactive oxygen species (ROS), widely reported as a major cause of cancer [32]. The capacity of cPa-SLN to neutralize ROS was also confirmed using the DPPH test, and as expected, was shown to be concentration-dependent (Table 2). The absorbance decay of the sample test was correlated with the absorbance decay of the control test, resulting in the percentage scavenging of free radicals translated as the antioxidant activity [23]. For the positive control (BHT), 78.11% scavenging of DPPH radicals was recorded at the highest-tested concentration (6.0 µg/mL); similar results were previously reported [23,33]. By plotting the obtained results, a linear regression ($y = 3.9814\,x - 3.9867$) with $R^2 = 0.9856$ was obtained, and the IC$_{50}$ was calculated as 195.08 µg/mL.

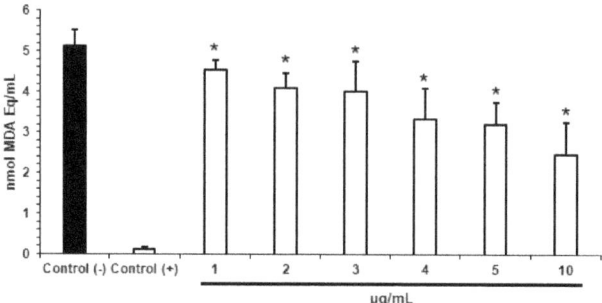

Figure 3. Effect of cPa-SLN (1, 2, 3, 4, 5 and 10 µg/mL) on the amount of malondialdehyde equivalents (MDA Eq.) produced in the presence of the free radical FeSO$_4$ inducers, performed in triplicate. Trolox and water were used as the positive and the negative control, respectively. Data are presented as mean ± SEM. * $p < 0.05$ when compared to the negative. One-way ANOVA with Dunnet post-test was applied.

Table 2. Evaluation of antioxidant activity (% scavenging of free radical DPPH) of perillaldehyde 1,2-epoxide from cPa-SLN.

µg/mL	AA%
1	0.59 ± 0.03
2	4.24 ± 0.02
3	7.39 ± 0.10
4	11.27 ± 0.05
5	14.93 ± 0.11
10	21.27 ± 0.12

From the results depicted in Table 2, increasing the concentration of lipid nanoparticles, the amount of the viable drug also increases, considering that more than 80% of the drug is loaded in the lipid matrices and is released in a time-dependent fashion (Figure 2). Our results confirm that cPa-SLN shows some antioxidant capacity (even if used at low concentration of particles) that can be exploited together with the antitumoral activity of perillaldehyde 1,2-epoxide in site-specific delivery. For a successful active targeting and site-specific delivery, the surface-modification of the particles is needed. The first step has been the streptavidin binding into cPa-SLN (cPa-SLN-S). Streptavidin is a protein purified from *Streptomyces avidinii*, showing high affinity for biotin, and is highly resistant to temperature variations, extreme pH values, organic solvents and proteolytic enzymes. It is usually recommended for the displaying of immobilized biotinylated antibodies [34,35].

To evaluate the capacity of cPa-SLN to bind streptavidin and produce the cPa-SLN-S complex, cPa-SLN were first diluted with PBS (1 mg/mL) and mixed, in different ratios, with aqueous streptavidin solution, as described by us [8], following the monitoring of z-Ave and ZP (Figure 4). While the amount of mAb successfully attached to biotin and then to the surface of cationic SLN could not be directly quantified, the amount of streptavidin and biotinylated antibody was optimized by a stepwise monitoring of the z-Ave and ZP of the obtained complexes, as well as their immediate stability in PBS.

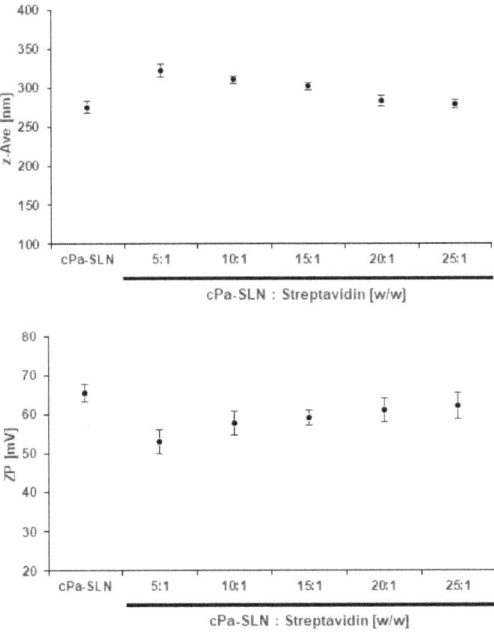

Figure 4. Variation on the mean particle size (z-Ave, upper panel) and zeta potential (ZP, lower panel) of cPa-SLN-S complexes obtained from different cPa-SLN—Streptavidin binding ratios. Results are given as a mean from three measurements of three independent experiments.

Although not statistically significant, a stepwise decrease in the z-AVE was shown with the increasing ratio of cPa-SLN—Streptavidin, i.e., the higher the amount of protein bound to the surface the higher the particle size (Figure 4, upper). The ZP decreased from 65.57 ± 2.23 mV (cPa-SLN) down to 53.06 ± 3.08 mV (5:1 w/w), which means that a stepwise decrease in the ZP was shown with the increasing amount of streptavidin. Although the decrease of ZP is associated with the increased risk of aggregation of particles in dispersion, the values remained well above +50 mV, ensuring a sufficient number of repulsive forces to maintain the electrostatic stability of the dispersions. Our results confirm the binding capacity of cPa-SLN to streptavidin. To further check the binding of the obtained complexes with the monoclonal antibody (cPa-SLN-S_{Ab}), 10 µg of biotinylated mAb was mixed with cPa-SLN-S complexes, obtained with ratios of 25:1, 15:1 and 10:1 in PBS. The z-Ave and ZP were again monitored (Figure 5).

The further increase in z-Ave with the antibody attachment up to 327.33 ± 6.21 nm and decreasing of ZP down to 51.04 ± 6.21 mV confirmed the binding and formation of cPa-SLN-S_{Ab} complexes. Again, the high ZP values ensure their stability in aqueous dispersion. Besides, proteins adsorbed onto the nanoparticles' surface can also provide some stereochemical stabilization, which was confirmed as no phase separation was seen.

For their further use as carriers in chemotherapy, the cytotoxicity of cPa-SLN-S_{Ab} (10:1 ratio) was checked in comparison to the non-surface modified particles (cPa-SLN) in MCF-7 cells (Figure 6). The cytotoxicity assay confirmed that the surface modification of the particles as the effect of the cationic lipid was attenuated, as shown by the increase in cell viability from 56.33 ± 1.99% when treated with cPa-SLN, to 63.30 ± 1.45% when treated with cPa-SLN-S_{Ab}, at the highest-tested concentration. We also observed that, at the lowest concentration, a drop of about 20% in cell viability occurred. This effect was attributed to the presence of CTAB in the formulations [36].

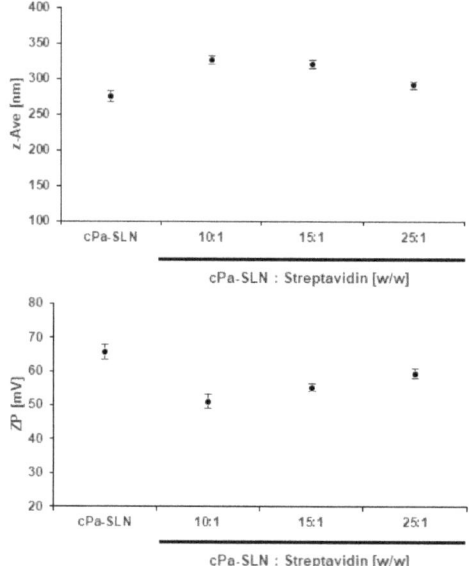

Figure 5. Variation on the mean particle size (z-Ave, upper panel) and zeta potential (ZP, lower panel) of cPa-SLN-S_{Ab} complexes obtained from the binding of the antibody with different cPa-SLN—Streptavidin binding ratios. Results are given as mean from three measurements of three independent experiments.

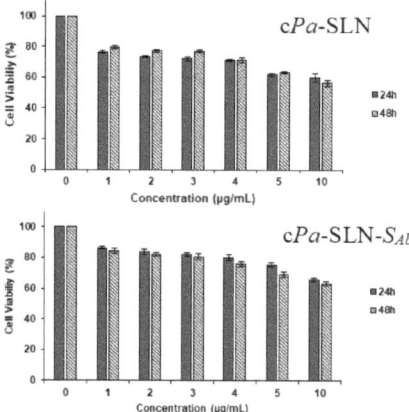

Figure 6. Evaluation of the cytotoxic activity of cPa-SLN and cPa-SLN-S_{Ab} in MCF-7 cell line using the MTT assay at 24 and 48 h.

4. Conclusions

The present study showed that the cytotoxic effect of perillaldehyde 1,2-epoxide against MCF-7 cell lines could be ameliorated when surface-modifying the particles with streptavidin. The particles exhibited some antioxidant capacity, attributed to the encapsulated monoterpene derivative. The cationic character of these particles provided a binding pathway via streptavidin to monoclonal antibody. The particles showed a modified release profile following the Korsemeyer–Peppas mathematical fitting. To further evaluate the affinity of mAb to HER2 receptors, the assessment of the targeting potential of the developed complexes and their cell internalization is planned, together with in vivo studies in a suitable animal model.

Author Contributions: E.B.S., S.B.S., A.Z., L.N.A. and P.S. contributed for the conceptualization, methodology, validation, formal analysis and investigation; E.B.S., S.B.S., A.Z., A.D., M.L., A.S., O.K.H., A.G.A., C.M., L.N.A., A.M.S. and P.S. contributed for the writing—original draft preparation; E.B.S., A.S., A.G.A., A.M.S. and P.S. contributed for supervision, writing—review and editing, project administration, resources and funding acquisition. All authors have made a substantial contribution to the work. All authors have read and agreed to the published version of the manuscript.

Funding: The authors wish to acknowledge the financial support from CNPq (Conselho Nacional de Desenvolvimento Científico e Tecnológico, from CAPES (Coordenação de Aperfeiçoamento de Pessoal de Nível Superior), and from FAPITEC/SE (Fundação de Apoio à Pesquisa e Inovação Tecnológica do Estado de Sergipe). E.B. Souto acknowledges the sponsorship of the projects M-ERA-NET-0004/2015-PAIRED and UIDB/04469/2020, receiving support from the Portuguese Science and Technology Foundation, Ministry of Science and Education (FCT/MEC) through national funds, and co-financed by FEDER, under the Partnership Agreement PT2020.

Conflicts of Interest: The authors declare no conflict of interest.

References

1. Doktorovova, S.; Santos, D.L.; Costa, I.; Andreani, T.; Souto, E.B.; Silva, A.M. Cationic solid lipid nanoparticles interfere with the activity of antioxidant enzymes in hepatocellular carcinoma cells. *Int. J. Pharm.* **2014**, *471*, 18–27. [CrossRef]
2. Doktorovova, S.; Shegokar, R.; Rakovsky, E.; Gonzalez-Mira, E.; Lopes, C.M.; Silva, A.M.; Martins-Lopes, P.; Muller, R.H.; Souto, E.B. Cationic solid lipid nanoparticles (cSLN): structure, stability and DNA binding capacity correlation studies. *Int. J. Pharm.* **2011**, *420*, 341–349. [CrossRef] [PubMed]
3. Doktorovova, S.; Silva, A.M.; Gaivao, I.; Souto, E.B.; Teixeira, J.P.; Martins-Lopes, P. Comet assay reveals no genotoxicity risk of cationic solid lipid nanoparticles. *J. Appl. Toxicol.* **2014**, *34*, 395–403. [CrossRef] [PubMed]
4. Fangueiro, J.F.; Andreani, T.; Egea, M.A.; Garcia, M.L.; Souto, S.B.; Silva, A.M.; Souto, E.B. Design of cationic lipid nanoparticles for ocular delivery: development, characterization and cytotoxicity. *Int. J. Pharm.* **2014**, *461*, 64–73. [CrossRef] [PubMed]
5. Fangueiro, J.F.; Calpena, A.C.; Clares, B.; Andreani, T.; Egea, M.A.; Veiga, F.J.; Garcia, M.L.; Silva, A.M.; Souto, E.B. Biopharmaceutical evaluation of epigallocatechin gallate-loaded cationic lipid nanoparticles (EGCG-LNs): In vivo, in vitro and ex vivo studies. *Int. J. Pharm.* **2016**, *502*, 161–169. [CrossRef]
6. Zakharova, L.Y.; Pashirova, T.N.; Doktorovova, S.; Fernandes, A.R.; Sanchez-Lopez, E.; Silva, A.M.; Souto, S.B.; Souto, E.B. Cationic Surfactants: Self-Assembly, Structure-Activity Correlation and Their Biological Applications. *Int. J. Mol. Sci.* **2019**, *20*, 5534. [CrossRef]
7. Jose, S.; Thomas, A.C.; Sebastian, R.; Shoja, H.M.; Aleykutty, A.N.; Durazzo, A.; Lucarini, M.; Santini, A.; Souto, E.B. Transferrin-Conjugated Docetaxel-PLGA Nanoparticles for Tumor Targeting: Influence on MCF-7 Cell Cycle. *Polymers (Basel)* **2019**, *11*, 1905. [CrossRef]
8. Souto, E.B.; Doktorovova, S.; Campos, J.R.; Martins-Lopes, P.; Silva, A.M. Surface-tailored anti-HER2/neu-solid lipid nanoparticles for site-specific targeting MCF-7 and BT-474 breast cancer cells. *Eur. J. Pharm. Sci.* **2019**, *128*, 27–35. [CrossRef]
9. Pereira, I.; Zielinska, A.; Veiga, F.J.; Santos, A.C.; Nowak, I.; Silva, A.M.; Souto, E.B. Monoterpenes Based Pharmaceuticals: A Review of Applications in Human Health and Drug Delivery Systems. In *Plant- and Marine-Based Phytochemicals for Human Health–Attributes, Potential and Use*; Goyal, M.R., Chauhan, D.N., Eds.; CRC Taylor and Francis: Boca Raton, FL, USA, 2018; pp. 85–130.
10. Campos, J.R.; Severino, P.; Ferreira, C.S.; Zielinska, A.; Santini, A.; Souto, S.B.; Souto, E.B. Linseed Essential Oil - Source of Lipids as Active Ingredients for Pharmaceuticals and Nutraceuticals. *Curr. Med. Chem.* **2019**, *26*, 4537–4558. [CrossRef]
11. Pereira, I.; Zielinska, A.; Ferreira, N.R.; Silva, A.M.; Souto, E.B. Optimization of linalool-loaded solid lipid nanoparticles using experimental factorial design and long-term stability studies with a new centrifugal sedimentation method. *Int. J. Pharm.* **2018**, *549*, 261–270. [CrossRef]

12. Zielinska, A.; Ferreira, N.R.; Durazzo, A.; Lucarini, M.; Cicero, N.; Mamouni, S.E.; Silva, A.M.; Nowak, I.; Santini, A.; Souto, E.B. Development and Optimization of Alpha-Pinene-Loaded Solid Lipid Nanoparticles (SLN) Using Experimental Factorial Design and Dispersion Analysis. *Molecules* **2019**, *24*, 2683. [CrossRef] [PubMed]
13. Zielinska, A.; Martins-Gomes, C.; Ferreira, N.R.; Silva, A.M.; Nowak, I.; Souto, E.B. Anti-inflammatory and anti-cancer activity of citral: Optimization of citral-loaded solid lipid nanoparticles (SLN) using experimental factorial design and LUMiSizer(R). *Int. J. Pharm.* **2018**, *553*, 428–440. [CrossRef] [PubMed]
14. Watkins, R.; Wu, L.; Zhang, C.; Davis, R.M.; Xu, B. Natural product-based nanomedicine: recent advances and issues. *Int. J. Nanomed.* **2015**, *10*, 6055–6074. [CrossRef]
15. Andrade, L.N.; Lima, T.C.; Amaral, R.G.; Pessoa, C.d.Ó.; Soares, B.M.; Nascimento, L.G.d.; Carvalho, A.A.; de Sousa, D.P. Evaluation of the cytotoxicity of structurally correlated p-menthane derivatives. *Molecules* **2015**, *20*, 13264–13280. [CrossRef]
16. Garcia, D.G.; de Castro-Faria-Neto, H.C.; Da Silva, C.I.; Gonçalves-de-Albuquerque, C.F.; Silva, A.R.; De Amorim, L.M.D.F.; Freire, A.S.; Santelli, R.E.; Diniz, L.P.; Gomes, F.C.A. Na/K-ATPase as a target for anticancer drugs: studies with perillyl alcohol. *Mol. Cancer* **2015**, *14*, 1. [CrossRef]
17. Chen, T.C.; Da Fonseca, C.O.; Schönthal, A.H. Preclinical development and clinical use of perillyl alcohol for chemoprevention and cancer therapy. *Am. J. Cancer Res.* **2015**, *5*, 1580.
18. Andrade, L.N.; Amaral, R.G.; Dória, G.A.A.; Fonseca, C.S.; da Silva, T.K.M.; Albuquerque Júnior, R.L.C.; Thomazzi, S.M.; do Nascimento, L.G.; Carvalho, A.A.; de Sousa, D.P. In Vivo Anti-Tumor Activity and Toxicological Evaluations of Perillaldehyde 8, 9-Epoxide, a Derivative of Perillyl Alcohol. *Int. J. Mol. Sci.* **2016**, *17*, 32. [CrossRef]
19. Andrade, L.N.; Severino, P.; Amaral, R.G.; Dória, G.A.A.; da Silva, A.; Alves, M.; Albuquerque Jr, R.L.C.; Luciano, M.C.S.; Pessoa, C.Ó.; Carvalho, A.A.; et al. Evaluation of cytotoxic and antitumor activity of perillaldehyde 1,2-epoxide. *J. Med. Plants Res.* **2018**, *12*, 590–600.
20. Doktorovova, S.; Kovacevic, A.B.; Garcia, M.L.; Souto, E.B. Preclinical safety of solid lipid nanoparticles and nanostructured lipid carriers: Current evidence from in vitro and in vivo evaluation. *Eur. J. Pharm. Biopharm.* **2016**, *108*, 235–252. [CrossRef]
21. Doktorovova, S.; Souto, E.B.; Silva, A.M. Nanotoxicology applied to solid lipid nanoparticles and nanostructured lipid carriers—A systematic review of in vitro data. *Eur. J. Pharm. Biopharm.* **2014**, *87*, 1–18. [CrossRef]
22. Pedersen, N.; Hansen, S.; Heydenreich, A.V.; Kristensen, H.G.; Poulsen, H.S. Solid lipid nanoparticles can effectively bind DNA, streptavidin and biotinylated ligands. *Eur. J. Pharm. Biopharm.* **2006**, *62*, 155–162. [CrossRef] [PubMed]
23. Souto, E.B.; Zielinska, A.; Souto, S.B.; Durazzo, A.; Lucarini, M.; Santini, A.; Silva, A.M.; Atanasov, A.G.; Marques, C.; Andrade, L.N.; et al. (+)-Limonene 1,2-epoxide-loaded SLN: evaluation of drug release, antioxidant activity and cytotoxicity in HaCaT cell line. *Int. J. Mol. Sci.* **2020**. submitted revised version.
24. Souto, E.B.; Muller, R.H. Lipid nanoparticles: effect on bioavailability and pharmacokinetic changes. *Handb. Exp. Pharmacol.* **2010**, *197*, 115–141. [CrossRef]
25. Jose, S.; Fangueiro, J.F.; Smitha, J.; Cinu, T.A.; Chacko, A.J.; Premaletha, K.; Souto, E.B. Predictive modeling of insulin release profile from cross-linked chitosan microspheres. *Eur. J. Med. Chem.* **2013**, *60*, 249–253. [CrossRef]
26. Aksoy, L.; Kolay, E.; Ağılönü, Y.; Aslan, Z.; Kargıoğlu, M. Free radical scavenging activity, total phenolic content, total antioxidant status, and total oxidant status of endemic Thermopsis turcica. *Saudi J. Biol. Sci.* **2013**, *20*, 235–239. [CrossRef]
27. Rigon, R.B.; Goncalez, M.L.; Severino, P.; Alves, D.A.; Santana, M.H.A.; Souto, E.B.; Chorilli, M. Solid lipid nanoparticles optimized by 2(2) factorial design for skin administration: Cytotoxicity in NIH3T3 fibroblasts. *Colloids. Surf. B Biointerfaces* **2018**, *171*, 501–505. [CrossRef]
28. Mahmoud, T.S.; Marques, M.R.; Pessoa, C.d.Ó.; Lotufo, L.V.; Magalhães, H.I.; Moraes, M.O.d.; Lima, D.P.d.; Tininis, A.G.; Oliveira, J.E.D. In vitro cytotoxic activity of Brazilian Middle West plant extracts. *Rev. Bras. Farmacogn.* **2011**, *21*, 456–464. [CrossRef]
29. Cavendish, M.; Nalone, L.; Barbosa, T.; Barbosa, R.; Costa, S.; Nunes, R.; da Silva, C.F.; Chaud, M.V.; Souto, E.B.; Hollanda, L.; et al. Study of pre-formulation and development of solid lipid nanoparticles containing perillyl alcohol. *J. Therm. Anal. Calorim.* **2019**, *10*, 1–8. [CrossRef]

30. Nita, L.E.; Chiriac, A.P.; Nistor, M. An in vitro release study of indomethacin from nanoparticles based on methyl methacrylate/glycidyl methacrylate copolymers. *J. Mater. Sci. Mater. Med.* **2010**, *21*, 3129–3140. [CrossRef]
31. Heydenreich, A.V.; Westmeier, R.; Pedersen, N.; Poulsen, H.S.; Kristensen, H.G. Preparation and purification of cationic solid lipid nanospheres–effects on particle size, physical stability and cell toxicity. *Int. J. Pharm.* **2003**, *254*, 83–87. [CrossRef]
32. Waris, G.; Ahsan, H. Reactive oxygen species: role in the development of cancer and various chronic conditions. *J. Carcinog.* **2006**, *5*, 14. [CrossRef] [PubMed]
33. Amaral, R.; Andrade, L.; Severino, P.; De Araujo, S.; Santos, M.; Dias, A.; Moraes Filho, M.; Ó Pessoa, C.; Carvalho, A.; Thomazzi, S.; et al. Investigation of the Possible Antioxidant and Anticancer Effects of Croton argyrophyllus (Euphorbiaceae). *Chem. Eng. Trans.* **2018**, *64*, 253–258.
34. Lu, X.-Y.; Wu, D.-C.; Li, Z.-J.; Chen, G.-Q. Chpater 7 - Polymer Nanoparticles. In *Progress in Molecular Biology and Translational Science*; Villaverde, A., Ed.; Academic Press: Cambridge, MA, USA, 2011; Volume 104, pp. 299–323.
35. Castner, D.G.; Ratner, B.D. Chapter 31—Proteins Controlled With Precision at Organic, Polymeric, and Biopolymer Interfaces for Tissue Engineering and Regenerative Medicine. In *Principles of Regenerative Medicine*, 3th ed.; Atala, A., Lanza, R., Mikos, A.G., Nerem, R., Eds.; Academic Press: Cambridge, MA, USA, 2019; pp. 523–534. [CrossRef]
36. Silva, A.M.; Martins-Gomes, C.; Coutinho, T.E.; Fangueiro, J.F.; Sanchez-Lopez, E.; Pashirova, T.N.; Andreani, T.; Souto, E.B. Soft Cationic Nanoparticles for Drug Delivery: Production and Cytotoxicity of Solid Lipid Nanoparticles (SLNs). *Appl. Sci.* **2019**, *9*, 4438. [CrossRef]

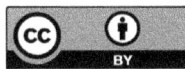

© 2020 by the authors. Licensee MDPI, Basel, Switzerland. This article is an open access article distributed under the terms and conditions of the Creative Commons Attribution (CC BY) license (http://creativecommons.org/licenses/by/4.0/).

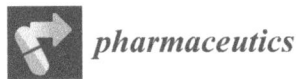

Article

Development of a Thymoquinone Polymeric Anticancer Nanomedicine through Optimization of Polymer Molecular Weight and Nanoparticle Architecture

Suhair Sunoqrot [1,*], Malek Alfaraj [1], Ala'a M. Hammad [1], Violet Kasabri [2], Dana Shalabi [2], Ahmad A. Deeb [1], Lina Hasan Ibrahim [1], Khaldoun Shnewer [3] and Ismail Yousef [3]

[1] Department of Pharmacy, Faculty of Pharmacy, Al-Zaytoonah University of Jordan, Amman 11733, Jordan; malek.fraaj@gmail.com (M.A.); alaa.hammad@zuj.edu.jo (A.M.H.); a.deeb@zuj.edu.jo (A.A.D.); linaibrahim9345@yahoo.com (L.H.I.)
[2] Department of Biopharmaceutics and Clinical Pharmacy, School of Pharmacy, University of Jordan, Amman 11942, Jordan; v.kasabri@ju.edu.jo (V.K.); danashalabi.ju@gmail.com (D.S.)
[3] Smart Medical Labs, Amman 11180, Jordan; khaldoun@clemjo.com (K.S.); info@smartlabs-jo.com (I.Y.)
* Correspondence: suhair.sunoqrot@zuj.edu.jo

Received: 3 August 2020; Accepted: 24 August 2020; Published: 27 August 2020

Abstract: Thymoquinone (TQ) is a water-insoluble natural compound isolated from *Nigella sativa* that has demonstrated promising chemotherapeutic activity. The purpose of this study was to develop a polymeric nanoscale formulation for TQ to circumvent its delivery challenges. TQ-encapsulated nanoparticles (NPs) were fabricated using methoxy poly(ethylene glycol)-*b*-poly(ε-caprolactone) (mPEG-PCL) copolymers by the nanoprecipitation technique. Formulation variables included PCL chain length and NP architecture (matrix-type nanospheres or reservoir-type nanocapsules). The formulations were characterized in terms of their particle size, polydispersity index (PDI), drug loading efficiency, and drug release. An optimized TQ NP formulation in the form of oil-filled nanocapsules (F2-NC) was obtained with a mean hydrodynamic diameter of 117 nm, PDI of 0.16, about 60% loading efficiency, and sustained in vitro drug release. The formulation was then tested in cultured human cancer cell lines to verify its antiproliferative efficacy as a potential anticancer nanomedicine. A pilot pharmacokinetic study was also carried out in healthy mice to evaluate the oral bioavailability of the optimized formulation, which revealed a significant increase in the maximum plasma concentration (C_{max}) and a 1.3-fold increase in bioavailability compared to free TQ. Our findings demonstrate that the versatility of polymeric NPs can be effectively applied to design a nanoscale delivery platform for TQ that can overcome its biopharmaceutical limitations.

Keywords: thymoquinone; polymeric nanoparticles; mPEG-PCL; anticancer nanomedicine; drug delivery

1. Introduction

Cancer is considered one of the leading causes of death worldwide and is responsible for millions of deaths annually [1]. Therapeutic success with conventional chemotherapeutic agents is complicated by their notoriously severe side effects, rapid clearance, and tumor relapse due to onset of multidrug resistance [2]. This has created a need to find alternative therapeutics and drug delivery systems that can eliminate cancer patients' tumor burden more effectively.

Throughout history, medicinal plants have been used to treat a wide range of diseases. Due to their structural diversity, natural products and their derivatives constitute a rich source of bioactive compounds with unique pharmacologic effects against various ailments including cancer [3]. *Nigella sativa* (black seed or black cumin) is an annual flowering plant endogenous to the Mediterranean region and parts of India and Pakistan [4]. Thymoquinone (2-isopropyl-5-methylbenzo-1,4-quinone; TQ) is the major constituent of the volatile oil of *N. sativa*. Since it was first isolated, TQ has been investigated for its therapeutic benefits such as antioxidant, anti-inflammatory, anti-diabetic, immunomodulatory, and anticancer effects, in both in vitro and in vivo settings [5]. Despite its prominent bioactivity, TQ has been faced with major biopharmaceutical challenges related to its poor aqueous solubility, hindering its therapeutic potential in vivo [6].

Nanotechnology has provided pharmaceutical scientists with versatile solutions that hold enormous promise to overcome the delivery challenges of hydrophobic bioactive natural products such as TQ [7]. Various types of nanocarriers have been explored in order to improve the therapeutic index, solubility, stability, circulation time, targeting efficacy, and bioavailability of poorly water-soluble drug candidates [8,9]. Several TQ-based nanocarrier systems have been reported in the literature. Many of these nanoscale formulations have been based on lipids, such as liposomes [10,11], solid lipid nanoparticles (NPs) [12], and nanostructured lipid carriers [13–15]. Inorganic NPs such as those based on gold [16] and silica [17] have also been investigated to improve the anticancer activity of TQ.

Polymeric nanocarriers represent a unique class of materials by virtue of their ability to be tailored for various biomedical applications depending on the choice of polymer and method of nanocarrier fabrication and drug incorporation. Fakhoury et al. reported the encapsulation of TQ into poly(styrene-*b*-ethylene oxide) NPs by flash nanoprecipitation [18]. The NP formulation exhibited equal cytotoxicity to MCF-7 cells and enhanced anticancer activity toward MDA-MB-231 cells compared to free TQ. Bhattacharya et al. utilized poly(ethylene glycol) (PEG) and poly(vinylpyrrolidone) to prepare TQ NPs by the solvent evaporation technique [19]. The NPs enhanced the anticancer activity of free TQ and mediated its anti-migratory effect on MCF-7 cells in vitro. TQ NPs were also able to protect tumor-bearing mice from cancer-induced systemic toxicity and hepatic damage. Another study by Soni et al. described the co-encapsulation of TQ and paclitaxel in poly(lactide-co-glycolide) (PLGA) NPs to achieve synergistic anticancer activity against MCF-7 cells [20].

In the present study, we aimed to design a polymeric NP formulation for TQ based on the copolymer methoxy poly(ethylene glycol)-*b*-(ε-caprolactone) (mPEG-PCL), and evaluate the NP formulation as a potential anticancer nanomedicine. Both PEG and PCL are FDA approved. In particular, PCL (alone or in the form of a PEGylated copolymer) has been widely used for the encapsulation of hydrophobic drugs due to its stability, controlled release properties, biodegradability, and biocompatibility [21–23]. mPEG-PCL can be synthesized with varying chain lengths of the biodegradable block (i.e., PCL) in order to modulate its physicochemical properties. It can also be used to prepare NPs with different architectures such as matrix-type nanospheres (NS) [24], reservoir-type (core/shell) nanocapsules (NC) [25], as well as polymeric micelles [26]. In this study, in order to reach an optimized NP formulation for TQ, mPEG-PCL NPs were fabricated using different PCL chain lengths in the form of matrix-type NS or reservoir-type NC. The different formulations were evaluated for various physicochemical properties and in vitro release kinetics. Antiproliferative assays were then conducted in human cancer cell lines to investigate the anticancer activity of the optimized NP formulation. A pilot pharmacokinetic study was also carried out in a murine model to evaluate the oral bioavailability of the optimized TQ NP formulation.

2. Materials and Methods

2.1. Materials

Tin(II) 2-ethylhexanoate (stannous octoate), ε-caprolactone (CL), methoxy poly(ethylene glycol) (mPEG) molecular weight (MW) 5000, Span 80, and thymoquinone (TQ) were obtained from Sigma Aldrich (St. Louis, MO, USA). Castor oil was provided by Philadelphia Pharmaceuticals (Amman, Jordan). Polysorbate 80 (Tween 80,) was purchased from RFCL Ltd. (New Delhi, India). Absolute ethanol, acetone, methanol (HPLC grade), isopropanol, formic acid, water (HPLC grade), and dichloromethane (DCM) were obtained from Fisher Chemical (Thermo Fisher Scientific, Waltham, MA, USA). Diethyl ether and dimethyl sulfoxide were provided by Tedia (Fairfield, OH, USA). Phosphate buffered saline (PBS) 10×, pH 7.4, was obtained from Biowest (Nuaillé, France). Ultrapure water (~18.2 MΩ·cm) was prepared using a Millipore Direct-Q 5UV system (EMD Millipore, Billerica, MA, USA).

2.2. Synthesis of mPEG-PCL Copolymers

mPEG-PCL copolymers were synthesized by ring-opening polymerization of CL as previously described [24,26], where mPEG served as the macroinitiator and stannous octoate as the catalyst to form mPEG-PCL block copolymers. PCL chain length was varied by controlling the mPEG:CL feed ratio (Table S1). ^{1}H-NMR in CDCl$_3$ (Bruker 400 MHz instrument, Billerica, MA, USA) was used to confirm the copolymers' structure and calculate the MW of the PCL block.

2.3. Preparation of TQ-Loaded NPs

Oil-filled core-shell TQ NC were prepared by nanoprecipitation as reported in our earlier publication [25]. The organic phase was a solvent mixture of acetone and ethanol (60:40, v/v) containing mPEG-PCL (25 mg), castor oil (150 µL), TQ (2.5 mg), and Span 80 (25 mg). The aqueous phase (10 mL) was composed of 0.2% Tween 80. The organic phase was added dropwise into the aqueous phase under moderate magnetic stirring and mixed overnight to evaporate the organic solvents and induce the formation of NC. Unencapsulated drug and excess excipients were removed by ultrafiltration (Pierce^{TM} Protein Concentrator, 100 kD molecular weight cut-off (MWCO), Thermo Scientific, Waltham, MA, USA) at 4000× g and 4 °C for 1 h (Hermle Z326K centrifuge, Wehingen, Germany), with repeated washing with ultrapure water twice. The final volume was completed to 10 mL with ultrapure water and the NP formulations were kept at 4 °C until further characterization. Matrix-type TQ NPs (NS) were prepared as described above without adding castor oil. The composition of the different TQ NPs prepared in this study is summarized in Table 1.

Table 1. Composition of thymoquinone nanoparticles (TQ NPs) prepared in this study.

Formulation	Organic Phase [a]			Aqueous Phase [b]
	Copolymer Code	Castor Oil (µL)	Span 80 (mg)	Tween 80 (% w/v)
F1-NS [c]	mPEG5K-PCL10.3K	-	25	0.2
F1-NC [d]	mPEG5K-PCL10.3K	150	25	0.2
F2-NS	mPEG5K-PCL18.5K	-	25	0.2
F2-NC	mPEG5K-PCL18.5K	150	25	0.2

[a] Composed of 5 mL acetone/ethanol (60:40, v/v); [b] Composed of 10 mL ultrapure water; [c] NS: nanospheres; [d] NC: nanocapsules.

2.4. Characterization of TQ NPs by Dynamic Light Scattering (DLS) and Transmission Electron Microscopy (TEM)

For DLS measurements, freshly prepared formulations were diluted 1:1 with ultrapure water and analyzed using a Nicomp Nano Z3000 particle size/zeta potential instrument (Particle Sizing Systems, Santa Barbara, CA, USA). Measurements were reported from at least three different batches of each NP. For TEM imaging, one drop of NP dispersion was placed on Formvar-coated Cu grids (300 mesh, Electron Microscopy Sciences, Hatfield, PA, USA). After 1 min, excess liquid was blotted with the edge of a filter paper, followed by staining with uranyl acetate for 1 min and removing the excess liquid with filter paper. Imaging was performed on a Morgagni 268 TEM (FEI, Eindhoven, The Netherlands) at an accelerating voltage of 60 kV.

2.5. High-Performance Liquid Chromatography (HPLC) Analysis

The amount of TQ loaded in NPs and the amount released during in vitro release studies was analyzed by HPLC. The setup was composed of a Finnigan Surveyor LC Pump Plus system (Thermo

Fisher Scientific, Waltham, MA, USA) equipped with an autosampler and a photodiode array UV detector. The mobile phase consisted of 0.1% formic acid, methanol, and isopropanol (50:45:5, *v/v/v*) at an isocratic flow rate of 1 mL min^{-1}. Elution was performed on a C18 UniverSil column (5 µm, 150 × 4.6 mm; Fortis Technologies Ltd., Cheshire, UK) and the detection wavelength was set to 260 nm. TQ serial dilutions (0.16–20 µg mL^{-1}) were prepared in the mobile phase and were used to construct the calibration curve, which was linear over the range of concentrations used (y = 218378x + 63037; R^2 = 0.99733). The method was validated according to the International Conference on Harmonization (ICH) guidelines. Limit of quantitation (LOQ) and limit of detection (LOD) values were found to be 5.33 and 1.76 µg mL^{-1}, respectively.

2.6. Determination of Drug Loading (DL) and Encapsulation Efficiency (EE)

For DL and EE determination, 0.1 mL of each freshly prepared NP dispersion was dissolved in 0.9 mL DMSO to ensure complete breakdown of the NPs. The samples were then diluted 1:1 in the HPLC mobile phase and analyzed as described above. The concentration of TQ was calculated based on a calibration curve of the peak areas of TQ standards versus concentration. Each measurement was performed in triplicate. DL and EE were calculated as follows:

$$DL\ (w/w) = \text{Weight of loaded TQ/Weight of polymer} \qquad (1)$$

$$EE\ (\%) = (\text{Weight of loaded TQ/Theoretical weight of TQ}) \times 100\% \qquad (2)$$

2.7. Characterization by FT-IR

FT-IR spectra were obtained using an IR Affinity-1 spectrometer (Shimadzu, Kyoto, Japan). KBr discs were prepared with powdered samples of TQ and mPEG-PCL, or TQ NPs which were lyophilized using a FreeZone 4.5 L Benchtop freeze dryer (Labconco Corporation, Kansas City, MO, USA).

2.8. In Vitro Release of TQ from TQ-NC

TQ release was investigated in phosphate buffer (pH 7.4) and acetate buffer (pH 5.0) to simulate physiologic and lysosomal/tumor microenvironment pH, respectively. All release media contained 0.5% *w/v* Tween 80 to ensure sink conditions [25–28]. For the release test, triplicate samples of freshly prepared NPs (1 mL) were each transferred to a dialysis bag with 12–14 kD MWCO (Spectrum laboratories Inc., Rancho Dominguez, CA, USA) and immersed in 30 mL release media in tightly closed glass vials. Samples were placed in an orbital shaking incubator operating at 37 °C and 100 rpm (Biosan ES-20, Riga, Latvia). At predetermined time intervals, 10 mL of release media was collected and replaced with an equal volume of fresh media to maintain sink conditions. Samples collected were kept at 4 °C until analysis. TQ concentration was measured by HPLC under the conditions described above. Results were expressed as % cumulative amount of TQ released versus time.

2.9. Release Kinetics

The following kinetic models were applied in order to elucidate the mechanism of TQ release:

$$\text{Korsmeyer–Peppas}: Q_t = k_{KP} t^n \qquad (3)$$

$$\text{Zero-order}: Q_t = Q_0 + k_0 t \qquad (4)$$

$$\text{First-order}: Log\ Q_t = Log Q_0 + k_1 t / 2.303 \qquad (5)$$

where t is the time, Q_t is the % cumulative amount of drug released at time t, k_{KP} is the Korsmeye–Peppas rate constant, n is the release exponent, Q_0 is the initial amount of drug released, k_0 is the zero-order rate constant, and k_1 is the first-order rate constant. Release data up to 60% cumulative release were fitted into each model.

2.10. In Vitro Antiproliferative Activity of TQ NPs

Antiproliferative activity was evaluated in various human cancer cell lines (MCF-7, PANC-1, and Caco-2) as well as a normal cell line (human dermal fibroblasts). All cell lines were obtained from the American Type Culture Collection (ATCC, Manassas, VA, USA). MCF-7, PANC-1, and Caco-2 cells were cultured in high glucose Dulbecco's modified Eagle medium (DMEM; Eurobio Scientific, Les Ulis, France). Fibroblasts were cultured in Iscove's modified Dulbecco's medium (IMDM; Eurobio Scientific, Les Ulis, France). All media were supplemented with 10% fetal bovine serum, 1% L-glutamine, and 1% penicillin/streptomycin. The cell lines were maintained at 37 °C in a 5% CO_2 atmosphere with 95% humidity. For the cytotoxicity experiments, cells were cultured in 96-well plates at density of 6×10^3 cells per well to ensure exponential growth throughout the experimental period and to ensure a linear relationship between absorbance and cell number when analyzed by the sulforhodamine B (SRB) assay. After 24 h of seeding, cells were treated with free TQ (from a 20 mM stock solution in DMSO) and TQ NPs (F2-NC, equivalent to 1.38 mM TQ dispersed in PBS) at concentrations equivalent to 3.12, 6.25, 12.5, 25, 50, 100, and 200 µM TQ for 72 h. At the end of the incubation period, 200 µL of ice-cold 40% trichloroacetic acid (TCA) was added to each well, left at 4 °C for 1 h, and washed five times with distilled water. The TCA-fixed cells were stained for 30 min with 50 µL of 0.4% *w/v* SRB in 1% acetic acid. The plates were washed four times with 1% acetic acid and air dried for 30 min. One hundred microliters of 10 mM Tris base solution was then added to each well, and the absorbance was recorded on a microplate reader (BioTek Instruments, Winooski, VT, USA) at 570 nm. Results were expressed as % cell viability compared to the control (untreated cells). Each experiment was performed in triplicate.

2.11. Pilot Pharmacokinetic Study of TQ NPs after Oral Administration

Thirty male Balb/c mice (8–10 weeks old) were housed in plastic cages in an air-conditioned room with free access to food and water and were fasted overnight prior to the experiment. On the day of the experiment, animals were divided into two groups and each group was administered a single dose of 6 mg/kg TQ either as suspension in ultrapure water or in the form of TQ NPs (F2-NC) via oral gavage. At 1, 2, 4, 6, and 24 h post-administration, three animals from each group were randomly selected and euthanized by diethyl ether, and blood (~1 mL) was collected from the jugular vein into heparinized plastic tubes. Blood samples were left to sit for 45 min at room temperature then centrifuged at 5500 rpm for 30 min at room temperature. Approximately 0.5 mL of plasma was collected into microtubes, and plasma samples were stored at −80 °C until further analysis. The animal protocol for this work was approved by the Animal Care and Use Committee of Al-Zaytoonah University of Jordan (decision no. 1/5/2019–2020). All work was conducted in accordance with the Helsinki guidelines for animal research [29] and all applicable Jordanian governmental rules and guidelines.

2.12. Analysis of TQ Plasma Levels by Liquid Chromatography-Tandem Mass Spectrometry (LC-MS/MS)

2.12.1. Instrumentation

The system consisted of a Shimadzu LCMS-8030 quadrupole mass spectrometer (Kyoto, Japan) equipped with an electrospray ionization (ESI) source, and a Shimadzu Prominence 30A Ultra-Fast Liquid Chromatography system composed of a system controller, degasser, binary pump and auto-sampler. Samples were eluted on a C8 column (5 µm, 50 × 2.1 mm) coupled with a guard column (5 µm, 10 × 2.1 mm) at 20 °C. The isocratic mobile phase consisted of acetonitrile (ACN) and 0.2% formic acid (50:50, *v/v*) at a flow rate of 0.2 mL min^{-1} and an injection volume of 20 µL. TQ samples were ionized by the ESI source in negative ion mode (5.5 eV spray voltage). The dwell time was set to 50 ms and the probe temperature was 400 °C. Quantification was performed using multiple reaction monitoring (MRM) of the transitions at *m/z* 164.0→134.1.

2.12.2. Preparation of Calibration Curve Samples

TQ was dissolved in ACN to make a stock solution at 1 mg mL^{-1}. TQ working standard solutions were prepared by serial dilutions of the stock solution in the mobile phase. Calibration curve samples were prepared by spiking the appropriate TQ working standard solutions into blank plasma obtained from untreated mice to achieve concentrations from 2 to 1000 ng mL^{-1}.

2.12.3. Preparation of Plasma Samples

To 100 μL of plasma (spiked with calibration curve samples or plasma extracted from treated mice), ethyl acetate (1 mL) was added and vortex mixed for 30 s. The solutions were then centrifuged at 14,000 rpm, and the supernatant was separated, dried, and reconstituted in 100 μL of the mobile phase. Samples were then injected into the LC-MS/MS system to quantify the plasma concentration of TQ at each time point. Pharmacokinetic parameters including the maximum plasma concentration (C_{max}), time to achieve C_{max} (t_{max}), plasma half-life ($t_{1/2}$), and the area under the curve ($AUC_{0\to\infty}$) were deduced from the plasma concentration versus time plots using Graphpad Prism 6.0e. Plasma $t_{1/2}$ was determined by fitting the elimination phase of the plots to the first-order model.

2.13. Statistical Analysis

Results were analyzed using Graphpad Prism 6.0e. All values were reported as mean ± SD. Statistical differences were examined by one-way or two-way analysis of variance (ANOVA) as appropriate, followed by Tukey or Sidak's multiple comparisons tests, respectively, where $p < 0.05$ was considered statistically significant.

3. Results and Discussion

3.1. Preparation and Characterization of TQ-Loaded NPs with Varying Polymer MW and NP Architectures

mPEG-PCL copolymers with two different PCL chain lengths were synthesized in this study by controlling the mPEG:CL weight ratio during synthesis. The structure of the copolymers and MW of PCL was confirmed using ^{1}H-NMR (Figure S1) by relying on the relative integration ratios between the proton peaks referring to the ethylene oxide repeating units and any one of the proton peaks of CL repeats [26]. Accordingly, when the feed ratio of mPEG:CL was 1:2, the MW of PCL was calculated to be 10,364 Da. A feed ratio of 1:4 produced a copolymer with a PCL MW of 18,506 Da. The two copolymers were referred to as mPEG5K-PCL10.3K and mPEG5K-PCL18.5K, respectively (Table S1).

mPEG-PCL copolymers were employed to fabricate TQ-loaded NPs by the nanoprecipitation technique. An overview of the NP preparation process is presented in Figure 1. This technique is typically used to fabricate matrix-type NPs where the loaded drug becomes entrapped within the polymer matrix as the organic phase is slowly added to the aqueous phase. The method can be adapted to produce reservoir-type NPs by incorporating oils in the organic phase [30]. With the appropriate combination of lipophilic and hydrophilic surfactants in the organic and aqueous phases, respectively, the procedure can lead to the formation of drug-loaded NPs with a core/shell architecture where the drug becomes entrapped in the oil core [31,32]. Various vegetable oils and triglycerides may be employed to form oil-cored NC [32]. In this study, castor oil was used as it has previously demonstrated superior ability to solubilize various polyphenolic and aromatic drug molecules during NC formation [25,33,34].

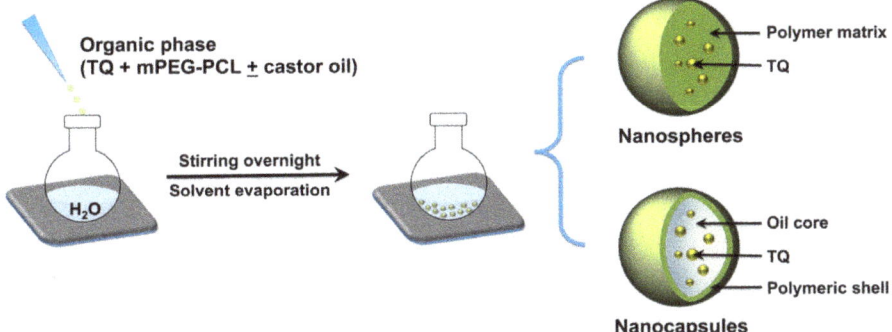

Figure 1. Overview of TQ NP fabrication by nanoprecipitation using mPEG-PCL. Different formulations were prepared by varying the MW of the PCL block with or without the addition of castor oil to the organic phase, which resulted in the formation of matrix-like nanospheres (NS) or reservoir-type nanocapsules (NC) with an oil-filled core and a polymeric shell.

The different NP formulations were characterized in terms of particle size, polydispersity, zeta potential, and drug loading efficiency (Figure 2 and Table S2). As shown in Figure 2A, particle size of the formulations was not impacted by the PCL MW, rather it showed strong dependence on the NP architecture. While both NS formulations F1-NS and F2-NS exhibited a similar particle size of 72 nm, the NC formulations F1-NC and F2-NC were significantly larger ($p < 0.001$) with an average particle size of 130 and 117 nm, respectively. Since the only difference between NS and NC formulations was the addition of castor oil, the increase in particle size may be attributed to the oil core–polymer shell architecture of NC. PDI values were used as an indicator of NP homogeneity in terms of size. As can be seen in Figure 2B, NC formulations were associated with PDI values of 0.17 and 0.16 for F1-NC and F2-NC, respectively. The NS formulations were significantly more polydisperse ($p < 0.05$) with average PDI values of 0.26 for both F1-NS and F2-NS. These findings are consistent with a previous report from our group using a similar combination of polymers, surfactants, and oil [25], and further confirm the ability of the NC architecture to produce highly monodisperse NPs. The zeta potential values for all formulations were partially negative and ranged between −9.2 to −14.2 mV (Figure 2C). Although the magnitude of the surface charge may not seem sufficient to impart colloidal stability, the presence of the PEG corona on the NP surface can effectively maintain steric stability and prevent NP aggregation, as evidenced by results from a previously reported stability study using a similar NP platform [25]. Moreover, the MW for PEG used in this study was 5000, which is within the MW range typically employed to achieve effective anti-fouling for nanocarriers [35].

The drug loading capacity of TQ NPs was found to be highly dependent on the NP architecture, while no difference in loading was observed between NPs with the same PCL MW (Figure 2D). NC formulations F1-NC and F2-NC were able to achieve 60.1 and 58.7% loading efficiencies, respectively, which were 2.5 and 2.2 times higher than the loading efficiencies obtained with F1-NS and F2-NS (24.0 and 26.3%, respectively). Again, the difference may be attributed to the presence of the oil-filled core in NC formulations, which has been shown to improve the NP loading capacity for lipophilic compounds compared to matrix-like NPs [33,36]. Based on these findings, it was concluded that the NC architecture was a more promising NP platform for TQ, and the NS formulations were excluded from subsequent investigations. TEM imaging of F2-NC (Figure 3A) showed a spherical morphology unlike F2-NS (Figure 3B), which appeared as polydisperse particles that were less uniform in shape. In addition, negative staining of the NC allowed the observation of the core/shell architecture, with the polymeric shell appearing as a light grey outer layer surrounding a darker core. On the other hand, F2-NS particles were characterized by a diffuse gray color with no discernible regions indicating their matrix-like architecture.

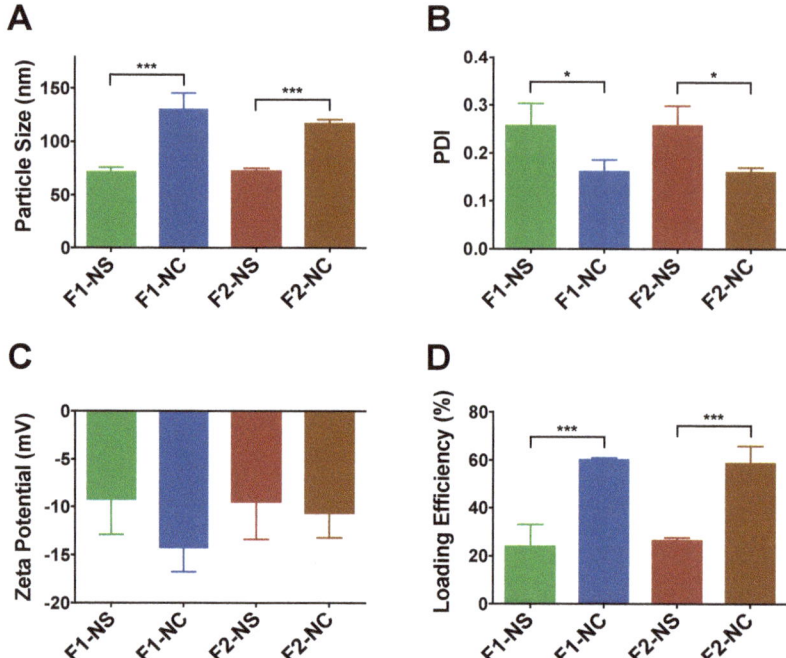

Figure 2. Characterization of TQ NPs prepared in this study. (**A**) Particle size of NC-based formulations F1-NC and F2-NC was 1.8 and 1.6 fold larger, respectively, compared to the NS-based formulations F1-NS and F2-NS due to the presence of the oil core; (**B**) NC-based formulations were associated with significantly lower polydispersity index (PDI) values, indicating greater monodispersity compared to their NS-based counterparts; (**C**) all NP formulations displayed partially negative zeta potential values; (**D**) the NC architecture is more favorable for TQ loading as evidenced by the significant increase in loading efficiency by 2.5 and 2.2 fold in F1-NC and F2-NC, respectively, compared to F1-NS and F2-NS. All results are presented as mean ± SD from at least three different batches of NPs. * $p < 0.05$, *** $p < 0.001$.

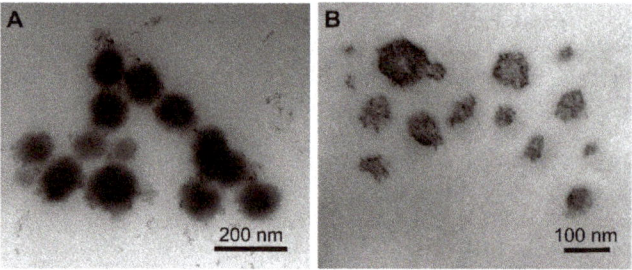

Figure 3. TEM images of (**A**) F2-NC and (**B**) F2-NS. F2-NC is characterized by a spherical morphology and core/shell architecture appearing as a dark core surrounded by a lighter outer layer, whereas F2-NS appeared as polydisperse matrix-like particles.

The NC formulations were further characterized by FT-IR spectroscopy. As shown in Figure 4, the FT-IR spectrum of TQ revealed characteristic bands corresponding to =C–H, C–H, and C=O stretching at 3050, 2970, and 1655 cm^{-1}, respectively. mPEG-PCL copolymers exhibited C–H stretching vibrations at 2950 and 2864 cm^{-1} which were attributed to the ethylene oxide repeats, and a sharp C=O stretching band at 1730 cm^{-1} corresponding to the carbonyl ester groups of the PCL repeats. Upon encapsulation of TQ to form F1-NC and F2-NC, several spectral changes were observed. A broad O–H stretching band appeared between 3700–3100 cm^{-1} in the NC formulations but was absent from the NS formulations F1-NS and F2-NS. This indicates the presence of hydrogen bonding interactions between the formulation components after adding castor oil which has three –OH groups. A similar observation was obtained when encapsulating the polyphenolic compound cirsiliol in castor oil-filled mPEG-PCL NC [25]. In addition, the =C–H stretching band of TQ was shifted from 3050 to 3014 cm^{-1} after encapsulation. This shift was accompanied by an increase in the intensity of C–H stretching vibrations between 3030–2780 cm^{-1}. The C=O bands of TQ and mPEG-PCL copolymers which originally appeared at 1655 and 1730 cm^{-1}, respectively, were also shifted to a single sharp band appearing at 1740 cm^{-1}. The spectral changes strongly indicate the compatibility of the formulation components enabled by intermolecular interactions such as H-bonding in addition to van der Waal forces.

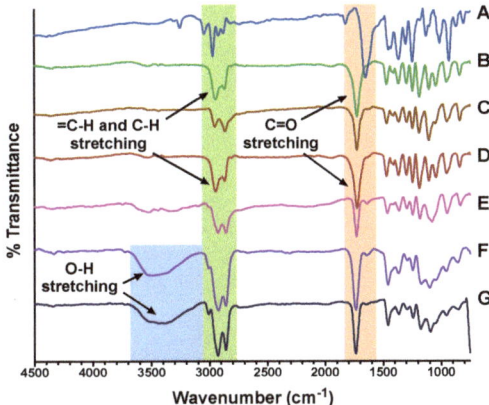

Figure 4. FT-IR spectra of (**A**) TQ, (**B**) mPEG5K-PCL10.3K, (**C**) mPEG5K-PCL18.5K, (**D**) F1-NS, (**E**) F2-NS, (**F**) F1-NC, and (**G**) F2-NC. TQ exhibited =C–H, C–H, and C=O stretching at 3050 cm^{-1}, 2970 cm^{-1}, and 1655 cm^{-1}, respectively. mPEG-PCL copolymers showed C–H stretching vibrations at 2950 and 2864 cm^{-1} attributed to the ethylene oxide repeats, and a sharp C=O stretching band at 1730 cm^{-1} corresponding to the carbonyl ester groups of PCL. The broad O–H stretching band appearing between 3700–3100 in the NC formulations (**F**) and (**G**) indicates the presence of hydrogen bonding interactions between the formulation components after adding castor oil.

3.2. Effect of PCL MW and pH of the Release Medium on TQ Release

In Vitro release of TQ from NC formulations F1-NC and F2-NC was investigated in PBS at pH 7.4 and in acetate buffer at pH 5.0 to mimic physiologic and lysosomal/tumor microenvironment pH, respectively. Samples were placed in dialysis membranes with MWCO 12–14 kD, which have previously been shown to allow free diffusion of small drug molecules with minimal effect on controlling drug release [25]. Samples were periodically withdrawn from the release media and were analyzed for TQ content by HPLC. The values were then used to construct the release profiles by plotting the cumulative % amount of TQ released from each formulation versus time. Release profiles of TQ from F1-NC at pH 7.4 and pH 5.0 are depicted in Figure 5A, whereas the release profiles corresponding to F2-NC at the same pH conditions are shown in Figure 5B. Both formulations resulted in the typical biphasic release profiles associated with polymeric delivery systems, with relatively fast release within the first 8 h and more sustained release up to 48 h. However, release was much faster in case of F1-NC, which achieved 86–90% cumulative release within the first 8 h in neutral and acidic media, respectively. In addition, the release profiles at the different pH conditions were superimposable. Conversely, TQ release from F2-NC was more sustained at pH 7.4, attaining 76% cumulative release within the first 8 h and 86% release after 24 h, which was accelerated in acidic media to reach 94 and 99% after 8 and 24 h, respectively. The difference in release kinetics was most likely attributed to the difference in MW of the biodegradable PCL. In the case of F1-NC, which was prepared using mPEG5K-PCL10.3K, the degradation of the PCL chains was relatively fast, even at neutral pH, resulting in a release profile similar to that obtained at pH 5.0. On the other hand, F2-NC prepared using mPEG5K-PCL18.5K was able to achieve better control over TQ release at pH 7.4 and faster release at pH 5, which is more favorable for in vivo applications.

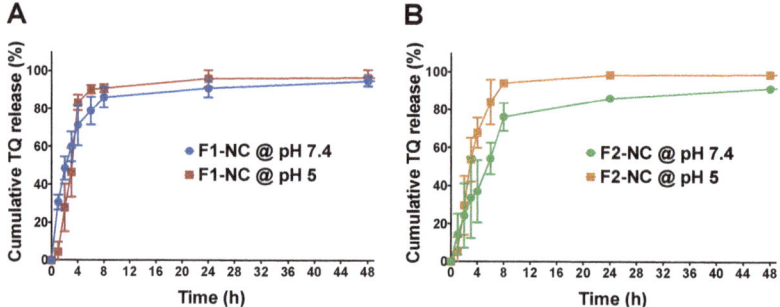

Figure 5. In Vitro release of TQ NPs conducted in phosphate buffered saline (PBS) (pH 7.4) and acetate buffer (pH 5.0). Results are presented as mean ± SD of cumulative % amount of TQ released from (**A**) F1-NC and (**B**) F2-NC up to 48 h. The PCL MW impacted the release kinetics. F1-NC with a shorter PCL chain achieved 86–90% cumulative release within the first 8 h in neutral and acidic media, respectively. Conversely, TQ release from F2-NC with the longer PCL chain was more sustained at pH 7.4, reaching 76% cumulative release within the first 8 h and 86% release after 24 h, which was accelerated in acidic media to 94 and 99% at 8 and 24 h, respectively.

TQ release kinetics as a function of PCL MW and pH conditions were further examined by fitting the release data up to 60% cumulative release to various kinetic models typically applied in polymeric systems, such as the Korsmeyer–Peppas, zero-order, and first-order models. Kinetic parameters were calculated and were used to find the best-fit model for each formulation/condition in order to better understand the mechanism of drug release. As summarized in Table S3, the goodness-of-fit for each formulation and pH condition was found based on the value of the coefficient of determination (R^2). Both F1-NC and F2-NC were best fitted to the Korsmeyer–Peppas model when release was conducted at pH 7.4 and the zero-order model when release was conducted at pH 5.0. At pH 7.4, F1-NC was associated with a release rate constant k_{KP} value of 31.0, which was greater than k_{KP} for F2-NC (14.6). The difference in k_{KP} between the two formulations correlates well with the faster release kinetics observed in F1-NC compared to F2-NC. The value of the release exponent n was also used to elucidate the mechanism of TQ release from the NP formulations. When the Korsmeyer–Peppas model is applied to spherical particles, a value of $n = 0.43$ indicates drug release by Fickian diffusion. On the other hand, a value of n between 0.43 and 0.85 is indicative of anomalous or non-Fickian transport. In this case, drug release occurs through a combination of simple diffusion and polymer chain relaxation. A value of $n \geq 0.85$ indicates supercase II transport, where drug release is primarily governed by polymer relaxation [37,38]. In this study, the value of n for TQ NPs at pH 7.4 was found to be 0.6 and 0.7 for F1-NC and F2-NC, respectively, signifying a similar release mechanism: anomalous transport. This mechanism is expected from core/shell systems when the shell is comprised of a biodegradable polymer. In the context of this study, TQ release most likely began by diffusion away from the oil core and across the polymeric shell into the release medium, while the polymeric shell was undergoing degradation and chain relaxation, which was faster in the case of F1-NC due to the shorter PCL chain. Interestingly, a recent study from our group reported much slower release kinetics for the flavonoid cirsiliol from a formulation similar to F2-NC, with ~20% cumulative release achieved within the first

48 h, and ~40% release attained after 96 h [25]. The difference may be attributed to the relatively small size of TQ (MW 164.2 g/mol) compared to cirsiliol (MW 330.1 g/mol), which allowed it to diffuse out of the NC formulation more freely.

When release was carried out at pH 5.0, both formulations exhibited zero-order kinetics, indicating constant TQ release from the NC core. F2-NC was associated with a release rate constant k_0 of 24.2 h^{-1}, whereas k_0 for F1-NC was slightly lower (21.0 h^{-1}). However, the two release profiles were similar across all time points (Figure 5A,B). The observed similarity in release kinetics at pH 5.0 indicates that the low pH of the release medium caused an acceleration in the degradation rate of mPEG5K-PCL18.5K, resulting in a similar contribution to controlling TQ release as that of mPEG5K-PCL10.3K. Based on these results, F2-NC was chosen for subsequent biological assays, having shown better control over release kinetics and pH-sensitive drug release.

3.3. Antiproliferative Activity of TQ-Loaded NPs in Human Cancer and Normal Cell Lines

Several mechanisms have been proposed for TQ's anticancer effects in various cell lines and animal models [39]. TQ has been shown to exert its cytotoxic effects by modulating multiple cancer hallmarks such as proliferation, cell cycle progression, invasion and metastasis, tumor-induced inflammation, and induction of angiogenesis [7]. In this study, the optimized TQ NP formulation (F2-NC) was examined for its antiproliferative activity in order to verify its potential to serve as an anticancer nanomedicine. In vitro assays were conducted in cell culture monolayers to screen the anticancer activity of the developed formulation and form the basis for future studies involving mechanistic understanding of the anticancer effects in vitro and in vivo. Assays were performed on MCF-7, PANC-1, and Caco-2 human cancer cell lines, with human dermal fibroblasts serving as a normal cell line to determine the NP's anticancer selectivity. The blank drug-free NC formulation was previously tested against cancer and normal cell lines and was shown to be nontoxic [25]. Cells were incubated with various concentrations of free TQ and F2-NC for 72 h, followed by assessing cell viability via an SRB assay. As depicted in Figure 6, free TQ and TQ NPs exhibited a dose-dependent inhibitory effect on cancer cell growth and the concentrations needed to achieve 50% growth inhibition (IC$_{50}$) were in the micromolar range (Table 2). The following order of potency was obtained for both TQ and F2-NC: PANC-1 > MCF-7 > Caco-2.

In general, free TQ was approximately two-fold more potent than F2-NC, which may be attributed to differences in cellular uptake and intracellular release kinetics of TQ from F2-NC. Note that previously reported NP formulations of TQ did not always result in potentiation of its anticancer activity. For example, TQ-loaded PEGylated polymeric NPs were more effective in killing breast cancer cells compared to the free drug [19]. On the other hand, Fakhoury et al. reported that TQ NPs exhibited equal or more potent anticancer activity compared to free TQ depending on the cancer model [18]. Moreover, a recent study by Ramzy et al. described TQ-encapsulated polymeric NPs targeted to colon cancer cells where the NPs were significantly less potent than free TQ due to sustained drug release [40].

Anticancer selectivity for free TQ and F2-NC was determined by the selectivity index (SI), which was calculated by dividing the IC$_{50}$ value obtained in fibroblasts for TQ and F2-NC by the IC$_{50}$ obtained in each cancer cell line. As shown in Table 2, the NP formulation exhibited superior anticancer selectivity compared to free TQ, particularly in PANC-1 cells where the SI for F2-NC was found to be 64.0 compared to 6.7 for free TQ. These results indicate that despite the lower potency for F2-NC, it may be more effective therapeutically than free TQ due to the enhanced cancer cell selectivity. These results were consistent with a recent report by Shahein et al., where TQ-loaded mesoporous silica NPs improved the drug's targeting efficacy toward cancer cells by exhibiting low toxicity to normal cells unlike free TQ [41]. Having shown the highest potency and the greatest selectivity against PANC-1 cells, our in vitro findings strongly support moving forward with F2-NC as a nanomedicine against pancreatic tumors in a suitable in vivo model.

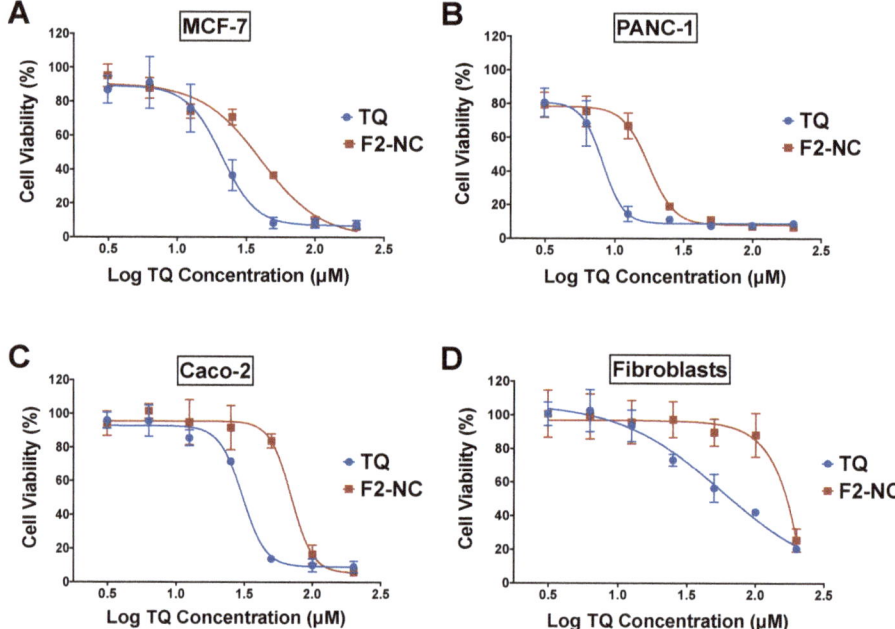

Figure 6. Antiproliferative activity of free TQ and the optimized TQ NP formulation F2-NC in (**A**) MCF-7, (**B**) PANC-1, and (**C**) Caco-2 human cancer cell lines, as well as (**D**) human dermal fibroblasts serving as a model normal cell line. Cells were incubated with various concentrations of TQ in its free or NP form in complete media for 72 h. Cell viability was measured via a sulforhodamine B (SRB) assay and expressed relative to untreated controls. TQ and F2-NC exhibited dose-dependent cytotoxicity with micromolar potencies across all cancer cell lines. Although free TQ was more potent than F2-NC, the latter was significantly less toxic to fibroblasts and was associated with a greater selectivity index.

Table 2. Summary of IC_{50} values and selectivity indices (SI) for TQ and F2-NC.

Cell Line	TQ		F2-NC	
	IC_{50} (μM)	SI [a]	IC_{50} (μM)	SI
MCF-7	20.5 ± 3.7	2.9	40.6 ± 2.1	27.9
PANC-1	8.8 ± 2.2	6.7	17.6 ± 1.2	64.0
Caco-2	30.4 ± 0.5	1.9	70.4 ± 0.2	16.0
Fibroblasts	58.9 ± 10.3	-	1129.5 ± 47.4	-

[a] Calculated by dividing the IC_{50} value obtained in human dermal fibroblasts by the IC_{50} value obtained in each cancer cell line.

3.4. TQ-Loaded NPs Are a Promising Strategy to Increase TQ's Oral Bioavailability

A pilot in vivo study was conducted in mice in order to evaluate the ability of the optimized TQ NP formulation to enhance the rate and extent of TQ absorption after oral administration. Animals were administered an oral dose equivalent to 6 mg/kg TQ either as aqueous suspension or in the form of F2-NC. At different time points, animals were euthanized and the plasma concentration of TQ was determined by LC-MS/MS. The resultant plasma concentration versus time profiles are shown in Figure 7, and the calculated pharmacokinetic parameters are summarized in Table 3.

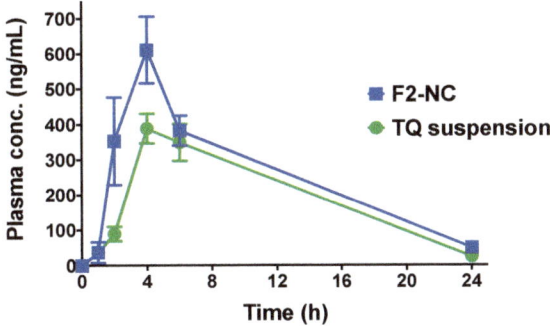

Figure 7. Plasma concentration versus time profiles following oral administration of TQ suspension or TQ NPs (F2-NC) to male Balb/c mice. Animals were divided into two groups (TQ suspension or F2-NC) and each group was given a dose equivalent to 6 mg/kg TQ via oral gavage. At 1, 2, 4, 6, and 24 h post-administration, three animals from each group were sacrificed and the plasma concentration of TQ was analyzed by LC-MS/MS to construct the plasma profile. Although both groups exhibited the same t_{max} of 4 h, F2-NC was able to achieve a significantly higher C_{max} compared to TQ suspension and a 1.3-fold increase in AUC, indicating superior bioavailability of the TQ NP formulation.

TQ suspension and F2-NC were both associated with a similar t_{max} of 4 h, indicating equal rates of absorption. However, F2-NC was able to achieve a significantly higher plasma concentration at 2 h ($p < 0.0001$). The NP formulation was also associated with a significantly greater C_{max} of 611.4 ng mL^{-1} compared to only 388.5 ng mL^{-1} for TQ suspension ($p < 0.001$). Consequently, F2-NC (AUC: 6069 ng h mL^{-1}) resulted in a 1.3-fold enhancement in bioavailability ($p < 0.05$) compared to TQ suspension (AUC: 4669 ng h mL^{-1}). Even though the elimination $t_{1/2}$ was slightly longer for F2-NC compared to TQ suspension (5.8 and 5.0 h, respectively), they were not significantly different. Taken together, these findings strongly indicate that F2-NC is readily absorbed from the gastrointestinal tract and can reach the systemic circulation to a greater extent compared to TQ suspension. This is largely attributed to the increased solubility of TQ when formulated as F2-NC compared to the poorly soluble free drug, consistent with previous reports involving TQ NP formulations [12–14]. Enhancing the solubility of hydrophobic drug molecules has been a leading motivation for pharmaceutical applications of nanotechnology. Based on the modest difference in $t_{1/2}$, it is likely that TQ is liberated from F2-NC during oral absorption and reaches the systemic circulation in its free form, resulting in similar elimination kinetics as TQ suspension.

Table 3. Pharmacokinetic parameters following oral administration of TQ suspension and F2-NC. Results are presented as mean ± SD ($n = 3$).

Parameter	TQ Suspension	F2-NC
C_{max} (ng mL^{-1})	388.5 ± 41.5	611.4 ± 94.9
t_{max} (h)	4.0	4.0
$t_{1/2}$ (h)	5.0	5.8
AUC$_{0\to\infty}$ (ng h mL^{-1})	4669 ± 508	6069 ± 492

4. Conclusions

In this study, we showed that NPs based on the biodegradable copolymer mPEG-PCL could be effectively tailored to design a nanoscale delivery system for the bioactive compound TQ. The optimal TQ NP formulation was found to be in the form of castor oil-filled NC based on the mPEG-PCL copolymer with the relatively larger PCL MW (F2-NC). F2-NC was associated with a monodisperse particle size, very good loading efficiency, spherical morphology, and sustained release properties. Even though the NC formulation exhibited lower anticancer potency compared to the free drug, it was associated with significantly greater selectivity, supporting its utility as an anticancer nanomedicine, particularly against pancreatic cancer where it showed the best selectivity. Preliminary pharmacokinetic evaluation in mice revealed an enhancement in oral bioavailability for F2-NC compared to free TQ, signifying its ability to enhance the biopharmaceutical properties of TQ.

Supplementary Materials: The following are available online at http://www.mdpi.com/1999-4923/12/9/811/s1, Figure S1: ^{1}H-NMR spectra of mPEG-PCL copolymers, Table S1: Characterization of the copolymers synthesized in this study, Table S2: Characterization of TQ NPs prepared in this study, and Table S3: Kinetic parameters for TQ release from F1-NC and F2-NC.

Author Contributions: Conceptualization, S.S. and A.M.H.; methodology, S.S., A.M.H., A.A.D. and K.S.; validation, S.S., A.M.H., V.K., A.A.D., and K.S.; formal analysis, S.S.; investigation, S.S., M.A., D.S., A.A.D. and K.S.; resources, S.S., V.K. and K.S.; data curation, M.A., D.S., L.H.I. and I.Y.; writing—original draft preparation, S.S., A.M.H., D.S. and K.S.; writing—review and editing, S.S., A.M.H., V.K. and A.A.D.; visualization, S.S.; supervision, S.S., A.M.H. and K.S.; project administration, S.S.; funding acquisition, S.S. All authors have read and agreed to the published version of the manuscript.

Funding: This research was funded by Al-Zaytoonah University of Jordan, grant no. 15/28/2017–2018.

Acknowledgments: The authors thank Doa'a Qattan from the University of Jordan, School of Medicine for assistance with TEM imaging.

Conflicts of Interest: The authors declare no conflict of interest. The funders had no role in the design of the study; in the collection, analyses, or interpretation of data; in the writing of the manuscript, or in the decision to publish the results.

References

1. WHO Cancer Fact Sheet. Available online: https://www.who.int/news-room/fact-sheets/detail/cancer (accessed on 1 April 2020).
2. Schirrmacher, V. From chemotherapy to biological therapy: A review of novel concepts to reduce the side effects of systemic cancer treatment. *Int. J. Oncol.* **2019**, *54*, 407–419. [PubMed]
3. Majolo, F.; Delwing LK DO, B.; Marmitt, D.J.; Bustamante-Filho, I.C.; Goettert, M.I. Medicinal plants and bioactive natural compounds for cancer treatment: Important advances for drug discovery. *Phytochem. Lett.* **2019**, *31*, 196–207. [CrossRef]
4. Darakhshan, S.; Bidmeshki Pour, A.; Hosseinzadeh Colagar, A.; Sisakhtnezhad, S. Thymoquinone and its therapeutic potentials. *Pharmacol. Res.* **2015**, *95–96*, 138–158. [CrossRef] [PubMed]
5. Woo, C.C.; Kumar, A.P.; Sethi, G.; Tan, K.H. Thymoquinone: Potential cure for inflammatory disorders and cancer. *Biochem. Pharmacol.* **2012**, *83*, 443–451. [CrossRef]
6. Ballout, F.; Habli, Z.; Rahal, O.N.; Fatfat, M.; Gali-Muhtasib, H. Thymoquinone-based nanotechnology for cancer therapy: Promises and challenges. *Drug Discov. Today* **2018**, *23*, 1089–1098. [CrossRef]
7. Schneider-Stock, R.; Fakhoury, I.H.; Zaki, A.M.; El-Baba, C.O.; Gali-Muhtasib, H.U. Thymoquinone: Fifty years of success in the battle against cancer models. *Drug Discov. Today* **2014**, *19*, 18–30. [CrossRef]
8. Patra, J.K.; Das, G.; Fraceto, L.F.; Campos, E.V.R.; del Pilar Rodriguez-Torres, M.; Acosta-Torres, L.S.; Diaz-Torres, L.A.; Grillo, R.; Swamy, M.K.; Sharma, S.; et al. Nano based drug delivery systems: Recent developments and future prospects. *J. Nanobiotechnol.* **2018**, *16*, 71. [CrossRef]
9. Sunoqrot, S.; Hamed, R.; Abdel-Halim, H.; Tarawneh, O. Synergistic interplay of medicinal chemistry and formulation strategies in nanotechnology—From drug discovery to nanocarrier design and development. *Curr. Top. Med. Chem.* **2017**, *17*, 1451–1468. [CrossRef]
10. Mohammadabadi, M.R.; Mozafari, M.R. Enhanced efficacy and bioavailability of thymoquinone using nanoliposomal dosage form. *J. Drug Deliv. Sci. Technol.* **2018**, *47*, 445–453. [CrossRef]
11. Odeh, F.; Ismail, S.I.; Abu-Dahab, R.; Mahmoud, I.S.; Al Bawab, A. Thymoquinone in liposomes: A study of loading efficiency and biological activity towards breast cancer. *Drug Deliv.* **2012**, *19*, 371–377. [CrossRef]
12. Singh, A.; Ahmad, I.; Akhter, S.; Jain, G.K.; Iqbal, Z.; Talegaonkar, S.; Ahmad, F.J. Nanocarrier based formulation of Thymoquinone improves oral delivery: Stability assessment, in vitro and in vivo studies. *Colloid. Surf. B* **2013**, *102*, 822–832. [CrossRef] [PubMed]

13. Abdelwahab, S.I.; Sheikh, B.Y.; Taha, M.M.E.; How, C.W.; Abdullah, R.; Yagoub, U.; El-Sunousi, R.; Eid, E.E.M. Thymoquinone-loaded nanostructured lipid carriers: Preparation, gastroprotection, in vitro toxicity, and pharmacokinetic properties after extravascular administration. *Int. J. Nanomed.* **2013**, *8*, 2163. [CrossRef] [PubMed]
14. Elmowafy, M.; Samy, A.; Raslan, M.A.; Salama, A.; Said, R.A.; Abdelaziz, A.E.; El-Eraky, W.; El Awdan, S.; Viitala, T. Enhancement of bioavailability and pharmacodynamic effects of thymoquinone via nanostructured lipid carrier (NLC) formulation. *AAPS Pharmscitech* **2016**, *17*, 663–672. [CrossRef] [PubMed]
15. Ng, W.K.; Saiful Yazan, L.; Yap, L.H.; Wan Nor Hafiza, W.A.G.; How, C.W.; Abdullah, R. Thymoquinone-loaded nanostructured lipid carrier exhibited cytotoxicity towards breast cancer cell lines (MDA-MB-231 and MCF-7) and cervical cancer cell lines (HeLa and SiHa). *BioMed Res. Int.* **2015**. [CrossRef]
16. Rajput, S.; Puvvada, N.; Kumar, B.N.P.; Sarkar, S.; Konar, S.; Bharti, R.; Dey, G.; Mazumdar, A.; Pathak, A.; Fisher, P.B.; et al. Overcoming Akt Induced Therapeutic Resistance in Breast Cancer through siRNA and Thymoquinone Encapsulated Multilamellar Gold Niosomes. *Mol. Pharm.* **2015**, *12*, 4214–4225. [CrossRef]
17. Goel, S.; Mishra, P. Thymoquinone loaded mesoporous silica nanoparticles retard cell invasion and enhance in vitro cytotoxicity due to ROS mediated apoptosis in HeLa and MCF-7 cell lines. *Mater. Sci. Eng. C* **2019**, *104*, 109881. [CrossRef]
18. Fakhoury, I.; Saad, W.; Bouhadir, K.; Nygren, P.; Schneider-Stock, R.; Gali-Muhtasib, H. Uptake, delivery, and anticancer activity of thymoquinone nanoparticles in breast cancer cells. *J. Nanopart. Res.* **2016**, *18*, 210. [CrossRef]
19. Bhattacharya, S.; Ahir, M.; Patra, P.; Mukherjee, S.; Ghosh, S.; Mazumdar, M.; Chattopadhyay, S.; Das, T.; Chattopadhyay, D.; Adhikary, A. PEGylated-thymoquinone-nanoparticle mediated retardation of breast cancer cell migration by deregulation of cytoskeletal actin polymerization through miR-34a. *Biomaterials* **2015**, *51*, 91–107. [CrossRef]
20. Soni, P.; Kaur, J.; Tikoo, K. Dual drug-loaded paclitaxel–thymoquinone nanoparticles for effective breast cancer therapy. *J. Nanopart. Res.* **2015**, *17*, 18. [CrossRef]
21. Grossen, P.; Witzigmann, D.; Sieber, S.; Huwyler, J. PEG-PCL-based nanomedicines: A biodegradable drug delivery system and its application. *J. Control. Release* **2017**, *260*, 46–60. [CrossRef]
22. Dash, T.K.; Konkimalla, V.B. Polymeric modification and its implication in drug delivery: Poly-epsilon-caprolactone (PCL) as a model polymer. *Mol. Pharm.* **2012**, *9*, 2365–2379. [CrossRef] [PubMed]
23. Gou, M.; Wei, X.; Men, K.; Wang, B.; Luo, F.; Zhao, X.; Wei, Y.; Qian, Z. PCL/PEG copolymeric nanoparticles: Potential nanoplatforms for anticancer agent delivery. *Curr. Drug Targets* **2011**, *12*, 1131–1150. [CrossRef]
24. Sunoqrot, S.; Hasan, L.; Alsadi, A.; Hamed, R.; Tarawneh, O. Interactions of mussel-inspired polymeric nanoparticles with gastric mucin: Implications for gastro-retentive drug delivery. *Colloids Surfaces B* **2017**, *156*, 1–8. [CrossRef] [PubMed]
25. Al-Shalabi, E.; Alkhaldi, M.; Sunoqrot, S. Development and evaluation of polymeric nanocapsules for cirsiliol isolated from Jordanian *Teucrium polium* L. as a potential anticancer nanomedicine. *J. Drug Deliv. Sci. Technol.* **2020**, *56*, 101544.
26. Sunoqrot, S.; Alsadi, A.; Tarawneh, O.; Hamed, R. Polymer type and molecular weight dictate the encapsulation efficiency and release of Quercetin from polymeric micelles. *Colloid Polym. Sci.* **2017**, *295*, 2051–2059. [CrossRef]
27. Sunoqrot, S.; Abujamous, L. pH-sensitive polymeric nanoparticles of quercetin as a potential colon cancer-targeted nanomedicine. *J. Drug Deliv. Sci. Technol.* **2019**, *52*, 670–676. [CrossRef]
28. Sunoqrot, S.; Al-Debsi, T.; Al-Shalabi, E.; Hasan Ibrahim, L.; Faruqu, F.N.; Walters, A.; Palgrave, R.; Al-Jamal, K.T. Bioinspired polymerization of quercetin to produce a curcumin-loaded nanomedicine with potent cytotoxicity and cancer-targeting potential in vivo. *ACS Biomater. Sci. Eng.* **2019**, *5*, 6036–6045. [CrossRef]
29. Ashcroft, R.E. The Declaration of Helsinki. In *The Oxford Textbook of Clinical Research Ethics*; Emanuel, E.J., Ed.; Oxford University Press: New York, NY, USA, 2008; pp. 141–148.
30. Fessi, H.; Puisieux, F.; Devissaguet, J.P.; Ammoury, N.; Benita, S. Nanocapsule formation by interfacial polymer deposition following solvent displacement. *Int. J. Pharm.* **1989**, *55*, R1–R4. [CrossRef]
31. Mora-Huertas, C.; Fessi, H.; Elaissari, A. Polymer-based nanocapsules for drug delivery. *Int. J. Pharm.* **2010**, *385*, 113–142. [CrossRef]

32. Pohlmann, A.R.; Fonseca, F.N.; Paese, K.; Detoni, C.B.; Coradini, K.; Beck, R.C.; Guterres, S.S. Poly (ε-caprolactone) microcapsules and nanocapsules in drug delivery. *Expert Opin. Drug Deliv.* **2013**, *10*, 623–638. [CrossRef]
33. Klippstein, R.; Wang, J.T.W.; El-Gogary, R.I.; Bai, J.; Mustafa, F.; Rubio, N.; Bansal, S.; Al-Jamal, W.T.; Al-Jamal, K.T. Passively targeted curcumin-loaded PEGylated PLGA nanocapsules for colon cancer therapy in vivo. *Small* **2015**, *11*, 4704–4722. [CrossRef] [PubMed]
34. El-Gogary, R.I.; Rubio, N.; Wang, J.T.-W.; Al-Jamal, W.T.; Bourgognon, M.; Kafa, H.; Naeem, M.; Klippstein, R.; Abbate, V.; Leroux, F. Polyethylene glycol conjugated polymeric nanocapsules for targeted delivery of quercetin to folate-expressing cancer cells in vitro and in vivo. *ACS Nano* **2014**, *8*, 1384–1401. [CrossRef] [PubMed]
35. D'souza, A.A.; Shegokar, R. Polyethylene glycol (PEG): A versatile polymer for pharmaceutical applications. *Expert Opin. Drug Deliv.* **2016**, *13*, 1257–1275. [CrossRef] [PubMed]
36. Khayata, N.; Abdelwahed, W.; Chehna, M.F.; Charcosset, C.; Fessi, H. Preparation of vitamin E loaded nanocapsules by the nanoprecipitation method: From laboratory scale to large scale using a membrane contactor. *Int. J. Pharm.* **2012**, *423*, 419–427. [CrossRef]
37. Korsmeyer, R.W.; Gurny, R.; Doelker, E.; Buri, P.; Peppas, N.A. Mechanisms of solute release from porous hydrophilic polymers. *Int. J. Pharm.* **1983**, *15*, 25–35. [CrossRef]
38. Siepmann, J.; Peppas, N.A. Modeling of drug release from delivery systems based on hydroxypropyl methylcellulose (HPMC). *Adv. Drug Deliv. Rev.* **2001**, *48*, 139–157. [CrossRef]
39. Majdalawieh, A.F.; Fayyad, M.W.; Nasrallah, G.K. Anti-cancer properties and mechanisms of action of thymoquinone, the major active ingredient of *Nigella sativa*. *Crit. Rev. Food Sci. Nutr.* **2017**, *57*, 3911–3928. [CrossRef]
40. Ramzy, L.; Metwally, A.A.; Nasr, M.; Awad, G.A.S. Novel thymoquinone lipidic core nanocapsules with anisamide-polymethacrylate shell for colon cancer cells overexpressing sigma receptors. *Sci. Rep.* **2020**, *10*, 10987. [CrossRef]
41. Shahein, S.A.; Aboul-Enein, A.M.; Higazy, I.M.; Abou-Elella, F.; Lojkowski, W.; Ahmed, E.R.; Mousa, S.A.; AbouAitah, K. Targeted anticancer potential against glioma cells of thymoquinone delivered by mesoporous silica core-shell nanoformulations with pH-dependent release. *Int. J. Nanomed.* **2019**, *14*, 5503–5526. [CrossRef]

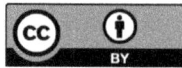

© 2020 by the authors. Licensee MDPI, Basel, Switzerland. This article is an open access article distributed under the terms and conditions of the Creative Commons Attribution (CC BY) license (http://creativecommons.org/licenses/by/4.0/).

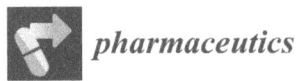

Article

π-Donor/π-Acceptor Interactions for the Encapsulation of Neurotransmitters on Functionalized Polysilicon-Based Microparticles

Sandra Giraldo [1,2,3], María E. Alea-Reyes [1,3], David Limón [1,3], Asensio González [1], Marta Duch [4], José A. Plaza [4], David Ramos-López [5], Joaquín de Lapuente [5], Arántzazu González-Campo [2,*] and Lluïsa Pérez-García [1,3,†]

[1] Departament de Farmacologia, Toxicologia i Química Terapèutica, Universitat de Barcelona, Avda. Joan XXIII 27-31, 08028 Barcelona, Spain; sandra.giraldo@ub.edu (S.G.); lyafalea@gmail.com (M.E.A.-R.); davidlimon@ub.edu (D.L.); gazulla53@gmail.com (A.G.); Lluisa.PerezGarcia1@nottingham.ac.uk or mlperez@ub.edu (L.P.-G.)
[2] Institut de Ciència de Materials de Barcelona (ICMAB-CSIC), Campus UAB, 08193 Bellaterra, Barcelona, Spain
[3] Institut de Nanociència i Nanotecnologia UB (IN2UB), Universitat de Barcelona, Avda. Joan XXIII 27-31, 08028 Barcelona, Spain
[4] Institut de Microelectrónica de Barcelona (IMB-CNM-CSIC), Campus UAB, 08193 Bellaterra, Barcelona, Spain; Marta.duch@imb-cnm.csic.es (M.D.); Joseantonio.plaza@imb-cnm.csic.es (J.A.P.)
[5] Parc Científic de Barcelona, Unitat de Toxicologia Experimental i Ecotoxicologia (UTOX-PCB), Baldiri i Reixac 10-12, 08028 Barcelona, Spain; ramos.lopez.david@gmail.com (D.R.-L.); qlapuente@gmail.com (J.d.L.)
* Correspondence: agonzalez@icmab.es; Tel.: +34-93-580-18-53
† Current address: Advanced Materials and Healthcare Technologies, School of Pharmacy, University of Nottingham, University Park, Nottingham NG7 2RD, UK.

Received: 3 July 2020; Accepted: 29 July 2020; Published: 1 August 2020

Abstract: Bipyridinium salts, commonly known as viologens, are π-acceptor molecules that strongly interact with π-donor compounds, such as porphyrins or amino acids, leading their self-assembling. These properties have promoted us to functionalize polysilicon microparticles with bipyridinium salts for the encapsulation and release of π-donor compounds such as catecholamines and indolamines. In this work, the synthesis and characterization of four gemini-type amphiphilic bipyridinium salts (**1·4PF$_6$–4·4PF$_6$**), and their immobilization either non-covalently or covalently on polysilicon surfaces and microparticles have been achieved. More importantly, they act as hosts for the subsequent incorporation of π-donor neurotransmitters such as dopamine, serotonin, adrenaline or noradrenaline. Ultraviolet-visible absorption and fluorescence spectroscopies and high-performance liquid chromatography were used to detect the formation of the complex in solution. The immobilization of bipyridinium salts and neurotransmitter incorporation on polysilicon surfaces was corroborated by contact angle measurements. The reduction in the bipyridinium moiety and the subsequent release of the neurotransmitter was achieved using ascorbic acid, or Vitamin C, as a triggering agent. Quantification of neurotransmitter encapsulated and released from the microparticles was performed using high-performance liquid chromatography. The cytotoxicity and genotoxicity studies of the bipyridinium salt **1·4PF$_6$**, which was selected for the non-covalent functionalization of the microparticles, demonstrated its low toxicity in the mouse fibroblast cell line (3T3/NIH), the human liver carcinoma cell line (HepG2) and the human epithelial colorectal adenocarcinoma cell line (Caco-2).

Keywords: π-donor/π-acceptor complexes; viologens; polysilicon microparticles; drug encapsulation; drug delivery; neurotransmitters

1. Introduction

The development of effective methods for drug encapsulation and release are topics of great importance because of the potential enhancement and prolongation of the overall efficiency of the drug as well as their controllable delivery in a target area. Different methodologies for drug encapsulation have been designed, such as: biocompatible complex microcapsules [1], modified nanocarbon materials [2] and mesoporous silica nanoparticles [3]. On the other hand, self-assembly monolayers (SAMs) and microfabrication techniques have been used to endow substrates of several properties to be applied in drug delivery. SAMs are a key tool in surface design of nanolayers for the bioactive coating of biomedical devices [4–6]. Different materials have been employed as substrates for the formation of monolayers, but gold and silicon [7–9] are the most widely used and studied, because of their biocompatibility and the ease of using thiol and silane chains, respectively, to be linked onto their surfaces to form well-organized monolayers. Moreover, microfabrication techniques allow the preparation of silicon-based devices with a great control of size, shape and monodispersity, properties that are important for biomedical applications and are a drawback of the chemical methods [10,11]. In this regard, microfabrication processes of silicon-based materials have provided polysilicon microparticles (Poly-Si μPs), which can be functionalized with a photosensitizer as singlet oxygen generators [12] or with lectins to obtain encoded Poly-Si μPs for tagging purposes [13,14]. Importantly, different studies have demonstrated their non-cytotoxicity using various cell lines [14,15]. Moreover, multi-material microparticles have been also microfabricated, showing interaction with different cell lines [16] or as innovative silicon-based intracellular sensors [17].

On the other hand, stimuli-responsive materials based on supramolecular complexes and their immobilization on surfaces can be highlighted as one of the potentials for drug encapsulation and sensing [18]. In this regard, bipyridinium salts, commonly known as viologens, are π-electron acceptor and redox-responsive compounds, which are able to generate π–π aromatic interactions with electron-rich groups such as amino acids [19] and neurotransmitters [20–22]. One of the better studied π-electron acceptor molecule, based on bipyridinium salts and widely employed to form catenanes and rotaxanes, is the cyclobis(paraquat-p-phenylene) ("blue-box") [23–25]. Moreover, viologens have attracted considerable interest not only for stimuli-responsive encapsulation methodologies, but also for other several applications including: building electrochromic devices [26], molecular electronics [27] and redox sensors [28]. Furthermore, the bipyridinium-based salts have also been used to functionalize silver nanoparticles [29], polymeric nanoparticles [30], microspheres [31], mesoporous silica [32], gold [33] and silicon surfaces [33,34], enabling the possibility of immobilizing bipyridinium salts on biocompatible surfaces for further microencapsulation and drug delivery applications. Thus, the combination of biocompatible microfabricated polysilicon-based devices with bipyridinium salts as hosts for a controllable encapsulation and release of π-donor biomolecules can open new opportunities for the delivery of drugs, whose physicochemical properties make their administration difficult. For this reason, in this work we explore the covalent and non-covalent functionalization of Poly-Si μPs with gemini-type amphiphilic bipyridinium salts used as host to assess the encapsulation and release of neurotransmitters, which present low stability in biological environments.

Neurotransmitters are π-donor biomolecules that play a pivotal role in communication between cells through signal transduction in living organisms [35]. Generally, an imbalance of these neurotransmitter levels could cause psychiatric and neurological disorders such as: depression, schizophrenia, Parkinson's and Alzheimer's diseases [36]. Therefore, ensuring adequate levels of neurotransmitters is necessary for preventing and treating undesired brain disorders. In this regard, advances in sensing methods for neurotransmitters' detection, and the development of carriers for their encapsulation and controllable delivery have been the focus of scientific interest in neuronanomedicine [37,38]. Thus, different carriers for neurotransmitters encapsulation have been described from liposomes [39], polymeric nanoparticles [40], mesoporous silica nanospheres [41] to amphiphilic anionic calix[5]arene micelles [42]. However, the further advancement of new responsive systems for controllable neurotransmitter delivery is still desirable.

Herein, this paper describes a new strategy to encapsulate and release neurotransmitters combining silicon-based microfabrication technologies and surface functionalization with bipyridinium salts. With this aim, the synthesis and characterization of four gemini-type amphiphilic bipyridinium salts **1·4PF$_6$–4·4PF$_6$** is first presented, which act as a host for the subsequent incorporation of the neurotransmitters: Dopamine (**D**), Serotonin (**S**), Adrenaline (**A**) and Noradrenaline (**NA**) (Figure 1). Moreover, a methodology for non-covalent and covalent functionalization of two polysilicon substrates, polysilicon surfaces (wafers) with a pattern of polysilicon microparticles on a thermal silicon oxide layer (Poly-Surfs) and square-shaped polysilicon microparticles (Poly-Si µPs, with **1·4PF$_6$–4·4PF$_6$** is developed for the further incorporation of the neurotransmitters. This incorporation, favored by π-donor/π-acceptor interactions between the neurotransmitters and the immobilized tetracationic hosts, is characterized by contact angle measurements. Furthermore, the quantification of **A** encapsulated and released using the non-covalent and covalent functionalization of microparticles with **1·4PF$_6$** and **4·4PF$_6$**, respectively, is studied using high-performance liquid chromatography (HPLC). Finally, the toxicity of **1·4PF$_6$** was determined as model of the bipyridinium salts used, performing cytotoxicity and genotoxicity studies in three different cell lines.

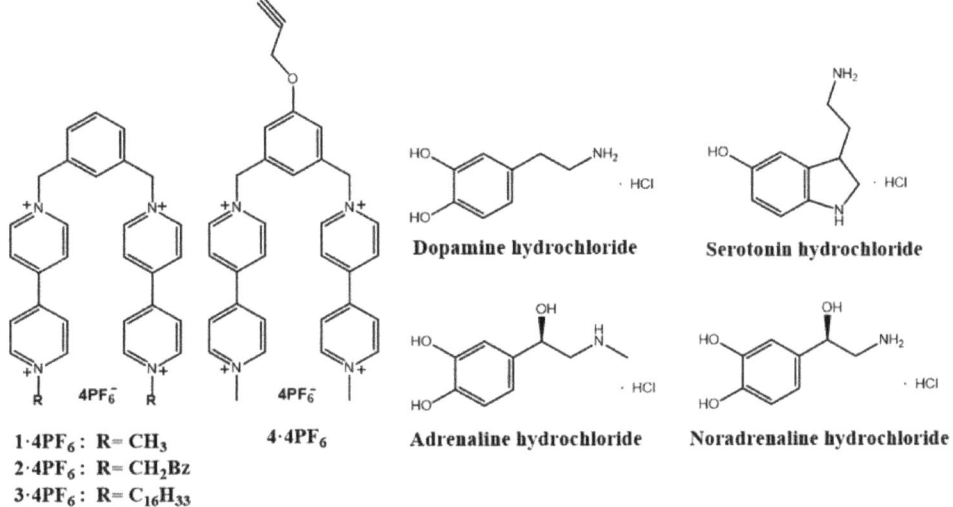

Figure 1. Bipyridinium salts **1·4PF$_6$–4·4PF$_6$** and neurotransmitters: dopamine hydrochloride (**D**), serotonin hydrochloride (**S**), adrenaline hydrochloride (**A**) and noradrenaline hydrochloride (**NA**).

2. Materials and Methods

2.1. Materials

Solvents: Acetonitrile (CH$_3$CN), dichloromethane (DCM), dimethyl sulfoxide (DMSO), dimethyl sulfoxide-d$_6$ ((CD$_3$)$_2$SO), N,N'-dimethylformamide (DMF) and nitromethane (CH$_3$NO$_2$) were purchased from Merck. Diethyl ether (Et$_2$O) was purchased from Carlo Erba and methanol-d$_4$ (CD$_3$OD) was purchased from Eurisotop.

Reagents: 1-Bromohexadecane, 1,3-bis(bromomethyl)benzene, 4,4'-bipyridine, adrenaline hydrochloride (**A**), 20% ammonia (NH$_3$), ammonium acetate (CH$_3$COONH$_4$), ammonium hexafluorophosphate (NH$_4$PF$_6$), ascorbic acid, benzyl bromide (BzBr), dopamine hydrochloride (**D**), 30% hydrogen peroxide (H$_2$O$_2$), iodomethane (MeI), noradrenaline hydrochloride (**NA**) and potassium iodide (KI) were purchased from Merck. 98% Sulfuric acid (H$_2$SO$_4$) was purchased from Scharlau and serotonin hydrochloride (**S**) was purchased from Alfa Aesar.

Compound **5**, the bipyridinium salt **2·4PF$_6$**, *N*-methyl-4,4′-bipyridinium iodide and 1,3-dibromomethyl-5-propargyloxy benzene were synthesized following reported procedures [25,43–45]. The fabrication process of both polysilicon substrates has previously been reported [12,46]. Neurotransmitter solutions were always freshly prepared and used immediately after their preparation as well as protected from the light.

2.2. Instrumentation

Melting points were measured by CTP-MP 300 hot-plate apparatus with ASTM 2C thermometer using crystal capillaries purchased from Afora. ^{1}H NMR: Varian Gemini 300 (300 MHz), and Varian Mercury 400 spectrometers (400 MHz) from *Centres Científics i Tecnològics de la Universitat de Barcelona* (CCiT-UB) and a Bruker Avance-400 spectrometer (400 MHz) from *Servei de Ressonància Magnètica Nuclear de la Universitat Autònoma de Barcelona* (SeRMN-UAB) service were employed. ^{13}C NMR: Varian Mercury 400 (400 MHz) from CCiT-UB and Bruker Avance-400 spectrometer (400 MHz) from SeRMN-UAB were used. NMR spectra were determined in (CD$_3$)$_2$SO or CD$_3$OD and the chemical shifts are expressed in parts per million (ppm) relative to the central peak of the corresponding solvent. Matrix-Assisted Laser Desorption Ionization-Time of Flight Mass Spectrometry (MALDI-TOF-MS) analyses were performed using a Voyager-DE-RP (Applied Biosystem, Framingham, USA) mass spectrometer, and high resolution mass spectra (HRMS) were obtained by Electrospray (ESI) on a LC/MSD-TOF mass spectrometer (Agilent Technologies, Santa Clara, CA, USA) from CCiT-UB. MS analyses were operated in delayed extraction mode using 2,5-dihydroxybenzoic acid (DHB) as matrix. Infrared spectroscopy (FT-IR) spectra were collected on a ThermoNicolet Avatar 320 FT-IR spectrometer (Thermo Fisher Scientific, Waltham, MA, USA) in a range of 4000–400 cm^{-1}, in KBr pellets (sample at 1%) and on a Spectrum One spectrophotometer (Perkin Elmer, Waltham, MA, USA) using attenuated total reflectance (ATR) at room temperature in a range of 4000–400 cm^{-1}. UV-Vis absorption spectra were obtained using V-780 spectrophotometer (JASCO, Madrid, Spain) and UV-1800 spectrophotometer (Shimadzu, Kioto, Japan), using quartz cuvettes with a 1 cm path length. Absorption spectra were determined in (4:1) DMSO: deionized H$_2$O solutions. Fluorescence spectra were measured using a Varian Cary Eclipse (Agilent, Santa Clara, CA, USA) and quartz cuvettes with a 1 cm path length and 1 mL volume. Contact angles (θ) were measured in air with high purity deionized H$_2$O by a 3 μL drop using a contact angle goniometer (THETALITE 100 with the software OneAttension, Espoo, Finland), in order to determine the hydrophobicity of the modified surfaces. Values of the contact angle on at least three samples were measured to give statistical significance. Microwave synthesis was done in a Monowave-400 from Anton Paar (Graz, Austria). Elemental Analysis was determined using Thermo Carlo Erba Flash 2000 at London Metropolitan University. Particle counting was performed by using 10 μL of dispersed microparticles on deionized H$_2$O disposed on a Neubauer Chamber from Brand with 0.100 mm Depth and 0.0025 mm^2 square size. The HPLC system used consisted of a Waters 600 pump and injector, with an Autosampler (717 plus), a 2996 Photo Diode Array and 2475 Multi λ Fluorescence detector. This system was equipped with an *Atlantis* dC18 5 μm pore column (150 × 3.9 mm). The analytical methods used were previously validated. For the analysis of **A**, the mobile phase consisted of a mixture of deionized H$_2$O (Channel A), CH$_3$CN (Channel B) and CH$_3$COONH$_4$ (100 mM, pH = 5) (Channel C). The method used was an Isocratic with a proportion of Channel A:Channel B:Channel C (88:2:10%) at flow rate of 1 mL/min and injection volume (10 μL). Samples were monitored and further analyzed at absorption wavelengths of 260–280 nm and 479 nm and emission wavelength of 315 nm.

2.3. Synthesis and Characterization of Compounds Based on Bipyridinium Salts

Arbitrary assignment of the proton and carbon atoms of **1·4PF$_6$**–**4·4PF$_6$** is described in the Supplementary Information (Figure S1).

2.3.1. Synthesis of 1,3-Bis(1′-methyl-4,4′-bipyridiniummethylene) Benzene-Tetrakis (Hexafluorophosphate) (1·4PF$_6$)

A solution of **5** (1.0 g, 1.7 mmol) in CH$_3$NO$_2$ (45 mL) was added to a solution of iodomethane (1.4 g, 10.2 mmol) in CH$_3$NO$_2$ (4 mL). The mixture was heated at 70 °C for 48 h. After cooling down to room temperature, the solvent was evaporated under vacuum. The yellow residue was then dissolved in H$_2$O (20 mL), and a saturated aqueous solution of NH$_4$PF$_6$ (1.7 g, 10.4 mmol, 3 mL) was added. The suspension was kept under strong stirring until no further precipitation was observed. Then, the suspension was filtered off and the solid was washed with H$_2$O (30 mL) and dried under vacuum to afford **1·4PF$_6$** (1.5 g, 87%); mp = 245 °C. ^{1}H NMR (400 MHz, (CD$_3$)$_2$SO, 25 °C): δ 9.43 (d, J = 8 Hz; 4H, H-9, 9′, 15, 15′), 9.26 (d, J = 8 Hz; 4H, H-14, 14′, 20, 20′), 8.77 (d, J = 8 Hz; 4H, H-10, 10′, 16, 16′) 8.71 (d, J = 8 Hz; 4H, H-13, 13′, 19, 19′), 7.81 (s; 1H, H-2), 7.55 (m; 3H, H-4, 5, 6), 5.93 (s; 4H, H-7, 8), 4.41 (s; 6H, N–CH$_3$). ^{13}C NMR (400 MHz, (CD$_3$)$_2$SO, 25 °C): δ 149.9 (C-11, 12, 17, 18), 148.5 (C1, C3), 146.9 (C-14, 14′, 20, 20′), 146.1 (C-9, 9′, 15, 15′), 135.4 (C2), 130.8 (C5), 130.1 (C4, C6), 127.4 (C-13, 13′, 19, 19′), 126.4 (C-10, 10′, 16, 16′), 63.8 (C7, C8), 48.7 (N–CH$_3$). MALDI-TOF–MS m/z: 881.1 (30%) [M-1PF$_6$]$^+$, 736.2 (40%) [M-2PF$_6$]$^+$, 591.22 (100%) [M-3PF$_6$]$^+$. HMRS (ESI) m/z: [C$_{30}$H$_{30}$F$_{12}$N$_4$P$_2$]$^{2+}$ calc. 368.09, found 368.08. FT-IR spectrum (KBr, cm^{-1}): 2920–2850 ν(C–H) (alkane), 1641 ν(C=N) and 835 δ(C=C).

2.3.2. Synthesis of 1,3-Bis(1′-hexadecyl-4,4′-bipyridiniummethylene) Benzene-Tetrakis (Hexafluorophosphate) (3·4PF$_6$)

A solution of hexadecylbromide (2.1 g, 7.0 mmol) in DMF (40 mL) was added to a solution of potassium iodide (0.5 g, 2.8 mmol) in DMF (4 mL). The mixture was heated at 80 °C and then, **5** (0.4 g, 0.7 mmol) was added portion-wise. The mixture was stirred for 7 days. After cooling down to room temperature, the orange precipitate was filtered off and washed with CH$_3$CN (10 mL) and dried under *vacuum*. The residue was then dissolved in DCM (4 mL) and a saturated aqueous solution of NH$_4$PF$_6$ (0.5 g, 2.8 mmol, 1 mL) was added until no further precipitation was observed. The suspension was filtered off and the white solid was washed with H$_2$O (30 mL), filtered off and dried under vacuum to afford **3·4PF$_6$** (0.7 g, 85%); mp = 280 °C. ^{1}H NMR (400 MHz, (CD$_3$)$_2$SO, 25 °C): δ 9.41 (d, J = 8 Hz; 8H, H-9, 9′, 15, 15′, 14, 14′, 20, 20′), 8.72 (d, J = 8 Hz; 8H, H-10, 10′, 16, 16′, 13, 13′, 19, 19′), 7.78 (d, J = 8 Hz; 2H, H-4, 6), 7.60 (t, J = 8 Hz; 1H, H-5), 7.46 (s; 1H, H-2), 5.97 (s; 8H, –CH$_2$–), 2.09 (s; 4H, H-7, 8), 1.24 (s; 52H, –CH$_2$–), 0.85 (s; 6H, –CH$_3$). ^{13}C NMR (400 MHz, (CD$_3$)$_2$SO, 25 °C): δ 149.7 (C-11, 12, 17, 18), 148.7 (C1, C3), 146.4 (C-14, 14′, 20, 20′), 146.2 (C-9, 9′, 15, 15′), 135.2 (C2), 130.1 (C5), 127.5 (C4, C6), 127.2 (C-13, 13′, 19, 19′), 127.0 (C-10, 10′, 16, 16′), 63.4 (C7), 61.4 (C8), 31.7–22.9 ((CH$_2$)$_{14}$), 14.4 (CH$_3$). MALDI-TOF–MS m/z: 1156.6 (3%) [M-2PF$_6$]$^+$, 1011.6 (100%) [M-3PF$_6$]$^+$, 866.6 (30%) [M-4PF$_6$]$^+$. HMRS (ESI) m/z: [C$_{60}$H$_{90}$F$_{12}$N$_4$P$_2$]$^{2+}$ calc. 578.33, found 578.32. FT-IR spectrum (KBr, cm^{-1}): 2918–2851 ν(C–H) (alkane), 1642 ν(C=N) and 837 δ(C=C).

2.3.3. Synthesis of 1,3-Bis(1′-methyl-4,4′-bipyridiniummethylene)-5-propargyloxybenzene-tetrakis (Hexafluorophosphate) (4·4PF$_6$)

In a microwave tube (10 mL), N-methyl-4,4′-bipyridinium iodide (0.2 g, 0.6 mmol), 1,3-dibromomethyl-5-propargyloxybenzene (0.09 g, 0.3 mmol) and CH$_3$CN (5 mL) were added. The mixture was irradiated in a microwave oven at 130 °C for 10 min. After that, a brownish precipitated was obtained and the final suspension was centrifuged with CH$_3$CN (3 × 5 mL). The brown residue was then dissolved in H$_2$O (15 mL), and NH$_4$PF$_6$ (260 mg, 1.6 mmol) was added. The suspension was kept under stirring until no further precipitation was observed and filtered off. The pale-yellow solid was washed with H$_2$O (20 mL) and with Et$_2$O (2 mL), filtered off and dried under vacuum to afford **4·4PF$_6$** (0.3 g, 81%); mp = 250 °C. ^{1}H NMR (250 MHz, DMSO, 25 °C): δ 9.44 (d, J = 7 Hz; 4H, H-9, 9′, 15, 15′), 9.28 (d, J = 7 Hz; 4H, H-14, 14′, 20, 20′), 8.78 (d, J = 7 Hz; 4H, H-10, 10′, 16, 16′), 8.72 (d, J = 7 Hz; 4H, H-13, 13′, 19, 19′), 7.44 (s; 1H, H2), 7.26 (s; 2H, H-4, 6), 5.91 (s; 4H, H-7, 8), 4.83 (d, J = 2 Hz; 2H, O–CH$_2$–), 4.44 (s; 6H, N–CH$_3$), 3.59 (t, J = 2 Hz; 1H, CH$_2$–C≡CH). ^{13}C NMR (250 MHz,

DMSO, 25 °C): δ 158.1 (C5), 149.3 (C11, C17), 148.1 (C12, C18), 146.7 (C-14, 14′, 20, 20′), 145.9 (C-9, 9′, 15, 15′), 136.2 (C1, C3), 126.9 (C-10, 10′, 16, 16′), 126.2 (C-13, 13′, 19, 19′), 122.3 (C2), 116.1 (C4, C6), 78.9 (C13), 78.5 (–C≡CH), 63,0 (C7, C8), 55.8 (O–CH_2–), 48.1 (N–CH_3). HRMS (ESI) m/z: $[C_{33}H_{32}N_4O]^{4+}$ calc. 125.06, found 125.06. FT-IR (ATR) (cm^{-1}): 3253 ν(C–H) (alkyne), 3031–2982 ν(C–H) (alkane), 2127 ν(C≡C), 1634 ν(C=N), 1556 ν(C=C) and 819 δ(C=C).

2.4. Formation of π-Acceptor/π-Donor Complexes between 1·4PF$_6$–4·4PF$_6$ and Neurotransmitters: D, S, A and NA in Solution

For **1·4PF$_6$–3·4PF$_6$**, a solution of either **D** (0.2 mg, 1.1 μmol), **S** (0.2 mg, 1 μmol), **A** (0.2 mg, 0.9 μmol) or **NA** (0.2 mg, 0.9 μmol) in deionized H_2O (0.5 mL) was added to a solution of either **1·4PF$_6$** (4.2 mg, 4 μmol), **2·4PF$_6$** (4.8 mg, 4 μmol), **3·4PF$_6$** (5.6 mg, 3.9 μmol) in DMSO (2 mL). The mixtures were stirred at 25 °C for 24 h under dark.

For **4·4PF$_6$**, a solution of either **D** (0.9 mg, 5 μmol), **S** (1.1 mg, 5 μmol), **A** (1.1 mg, 5 μmol) or **NA** (1.0 mg, 5 μmol) in deionized H_2O (0.5 mL) was added to a solution of **4·4PF$_6$** (5.4 mg, 5 μmol) in DMSO (2 mL), being the final concentration for each component 2 mM. The mixtures were stirred at 25 °C for 24 h under dark.

2.5. Functionalization of Polysilicon Surfaces (Poly-Surfs) with Bipyridinium Salts 1·4PF$_6$–4·4PF$_6$, and Incorporation of D, S, A and NA

2.5.1. Cleaning and Activation Surface Protocol

The polysilicon surfaces were immersed in a freshly prepared piranha solution, H_2SO_4: H_2O_2 at a volume ratio of 7:3 (1.4, 0.6 mL, respectively) during 1.5 h at room temperature. Then, the substrates were rinsed with deionized H_2O (2 × 2 mL), dried with N_2 flow and immediately immersed in an alkaline mixture of NH_4OH: H_2O_2: H_2O, at a volume ratio 1:1:5 (0.3, 0.3, 1.4 mL, respectively) for 30 min. The substrates were rinsed with deionized H_2O (2 × 2 mL) and dried with N_2 flow.

2.5.2. Non-Covalent Immobilization of **1·4PF$_6$–3·4PF$_6$** and Incorporation of **D, S, A** and **NA**

The hydroxylated surfaces were immediately immersed in a solution of either **1·4PF$_6$** (2.1 mg, 1 mM), **2·4PF$_6$** (2.4 mg, 1 mM) or **3·4PF$_6$** (2.9 mg, 1 mM) in DMSO (2 mL) and were stirred at 90 rpm for 6 h. After the deposition time, the substrates were rinsed with DMSO (5 × 3 mL) and deionized H_2O (5 × 3 mL) and dried with N_2 flow. The functionalized substrates with either **1·4PF$_6$**, **2·4PF$_6$**, **3·4PF$_6$** were immersed in a solution of either **D** (0.8 mg, 2 mM), **S** (0.9 mg, 2 mM), **A** (0.9 mg, 2 mM) or **NA** (0.8 mg, 2 mM) in deionized H_2O (2 mL) and were stirred at 90 rpm for 24 h. After this time, the substrates were rinsed with deionized H_2O (5 × 3 mL) and dried with N_2 flow.

2.5.3. Covalent Immobilization of **4·4PF$_6$** and Incorporation of **D, S, A** and **NA**

The hydroxylated surfaces were immersed in a solution of 11-azidoundecyltrimethoxysilane (20 μL, 30.6 mM) in toluene (2 mL) and stirred at 90 rpm overnight, rinsed with toluene (2 × 2 mL) and EtOH (2 × 2 mL) and dried with N_2 flow. Then, the azido-functionalized surfaces were immersed in a mixture of **4·4PF$_6$** (4.3 mg, 1 mM), $CuSO_4$ (64 μg, 0.1 mM) and sodium ascorbate (0.8 mg, 1 mM) in EtOH: H_2O: DMSO at volume ratio (3 mL, 0.6 mL, 0.4 mL) and stirred at 90 rpm overnight at 40 °C. After this time, the substrates were rinsed with EtOH (2 × 4 mL) and deionized H_2O (2 × 4 mL) and dried with N_2 flow. The functionalized substrates with **4·4PF$_6$** were immersed in a solution of either **D** (1.9 mg, 2 mM), **S** (2.1 mg, 2 mM), **A** (2.2 mg, 2 mM) or **NA** (2.1 mg, 2 mM) in deionized H_2O (5 mL) and were stirred at 90 rpm for 24 h. After this time, the substrates were rinsed with deionized H_2O (2 × 5 mL) and dried with N_2 flow.

2.5.4. Control Surfaces with D, S, A and NA

The hydroxylated polysilicon surfaces used as control experiments were separately immersed in a solution of either neurotransmitter (2 mM) in deionized H_2O (2 mL) for 24 h. After this time, the substrates were rinsed with deionized H_2O (2 × 5 mL) and dried with N_2 flow.

2.6. Functionalization of Polysilicon Microparticles (Poly-Si µPs) with 1·4PF$_6$ and 4·4PF$_6$ and Incorporation of A

2.6.1. Cleaning and Activation Protocol of Poly-Si µPs

A total of 100 µL of a freshly prepared piranha solution (H_2SO_4:H_2O_2) at volume ratio of 7:3 (0.7 mL, 0.3 mL, respectively) was added to different microtubes containing 1.5×10^6 polysilicon microparticles. The suspension was incubated for 1.5 h at room temperature while stirred on a vortex mixer at 400 rpm and then centrifuged (13,500 rpm, 15 min), forming a pellet of microparticles, which were resuspended and washed with deionized H_2O (2 × 100 µL). The suspension was centrifuged (13,500 rpm, 10 min) forming a pellet of microparticles and the supernatant was removed. Then, 100 µL of a freshly prepared alkaline mixture of NH_4OH: H_2O_2: H_2O, at a volume ratio 1:1:5 (0.1 mL, 0.1 mL, 0.7 mL, respectively) was added to the pellet. After resuspending the microparticles, they were stirred on a vortex mixer at 400 rpm for 30 minutes. After this time, the suspension was centrifuged (13,500 rpm, 15 min) and washed with deionized H_2O (2 × 100 µL) and EtOH (100 µL), centrifuging (13,500 rpm, 10 min) after each washing step and removing the supernatant.

2.6.2. Non-Covalent Immobilization of 1·4PF$_6$ on Poly-Si µPs

A total of 100 µL of a solution of 1·4PF$_6$ (2.1 mg, 1 mM) in DMSO (2 mL) was added to the pellet of the hydroxylated microparticles. The microtubes containing the microparticles were stirred at 400 rpm overnight. After the deposition time, microparticles were sedimented by centrifugation (13,500 rpm, 10 min) and washed with DMSO (5 × 100 µL).

2.6.3. Covalent Immobilization of 4·4PF$_6$ on Poly-Si µPs

The hydroxylated microparticles were immersed in 100 µL of a solution of 11-azidoundecyltrimethoxysilane (10 µL, 15.3 mM) in toluene (1 mL) and stirred on a vortex mixer at 400 rpm overnight. The suspension was then centrifuged (13,500 rpm, 10 min), washed with toluene (2 × 100 µL) and EtOH (100 µL), centrifuging (13,500 rpm, 10 min) after each washing step and removing the supernatant. After that, to the azido-functionalized microparticles, 200 µL of a mixture of 4·4PF$_6$ (1.08 mg, 1 mM), $CuSO_4$ (0.032 mg, 0.1 mM) and sodium ascorbate (0.2 mg, 1 mM) in EtOH: H_2O:DMSO (0.5, 0.3, 0.2 mL) were added. The microtubes containing the microparticles were stirred on a vortex mixer at 400 rpm overnight at 40 °C. Then, the microparticles were sedimented by centrifugation (13,500 rpm, 10 min) and the supernatant was removed. The microparticles were washed with EtOH (2 × 200 µL) and deionized H_2O (2 × 200 µL), centrifuging (13,500 rpm, 10 min) after each washing step and removing the supernatant.

2.6.4. Incorporation of A in 1·4PF$_6$ and 4·4PF$_6$ Functionalized Poly-Si µPs

A total of 200 µL of an aqueous solution of A (2.64 mg, 2mM) in deionized H_2O (6 mL) was added to the suspension of polysilicon microparticles functionalized with 1·4PF$_6$ or 4·4PF$_6$. All microtubes (four microtubes for each 1·4PF$_6$ and 4·4PF$_6$, respectively) were stirred on a vortex mixer at 400 rpm for 24 h at room temperature. After this time, microparticles were sedimented by centrifugation (13,500 rpm, 10 min) and washed with deionized H_2O (3 × 200 µL), centrifuging (13,500 rpm, 10 min) after each washing step and removing the supernatant.

2.7. Quantification of A Incorporated in Poly-Si µPs by HPLC Determination

After the incubation of the functionalized microparticles (**1·4PF$_6$** or **4·4PF$_6$**) with **A**, the suspensions of the four microtubes were centrifuged (13,500 rpm, 10 min) and the supernatant of each microtube was kept. A total of 100 µL of each supernatant solution was diluted up to 1 mL with deionized H$_2$O (900 µL), considered as the final solution (**A$_{fin}$**). Moreover, 100 µL of the 2 mM solution of **A** in deionized H$_2$O were diluted up to 1 mL, with deionized H$_2$O (900 µL) being the initial solution (**A$_{in}$**). These **A$_{in}$** and **A$_{fin}$** solutions were analyzed by HPLC coupled to a fluorescence detector (λ_{exc} = 280 nm, λ_{em} = 315 nm). The retention time of **A** was 2.5 min and the area under the curve (AUC) of the retention peaks was measured. The amount of **A** incorporated was estimated using a calibration curve of **A** in a range of 0.18–7.21 × 10^{-4} mM in deionized H$_2$O.

In order to calculate the final amount of microparticles, they were suspended in 100 µL of deionized H$_2$O. A total of 10 µL of each suspension was deposited in a Neubauer chamber and images by optical microscope were collected.

2.8. Quantification of A Released from Poly-Si µPs by HPLC Determination

The microparticles functionalized with either **1·4PF$_6$:A** or **4·4PF$_6$:A** of the four microtubes used were collected in a single microtube and centrifuged (13,000 rpm, 10 min). A total of 200 µL of a solution of ascorbic acid (4 mM) in deionized H$_2$O (200 µL) was added to the precipitated microparticles with either **1·4PF$_6$:A** or **4·4PF$_6$:A**. The microparticles were then suspended by sonication (1 min) and the suspension was incubated for 20 min at room temperature without stirring. Afterwards, microparticles were sedimented by centrifugation (13,000 rpm, 10 min), and the supernatant was collected (release solution—T1). The release process with ascorbic acid was repeated and a second release solution (release solution—T2) was collected. The release solutions (T1 and T2) were analyzed by HPLC coupled to a fluorescence detector (λ_{exc} = 280 nm, λ_{em} = 315 nm). The retention time of **A** was 2.5 min and the area under the curve (AUC) of the retention peaks was measured. The amount of **A** released was estimated using a calibration curve of **A** in a range of 0.18–7.21 × 10^{-4} mM in deionized H$_2$O.

3. Results and Discussion

3.1. Synthesis of 1·4PF$_6$–4·4PF$_6$

In this work, four π-deficient bipyridinium salts (**1·4PF$_6$–4·4PF$_6$**) have been synthesized and characterized. These π-deficient salts were used as hosts in the non-covalent and covalent functionalization of polysilicon surfaces and microparticles for the subsequent encapsulation and release of π-excessive neurotransmitters. These π-deficient systems are composed of two bipyridinium units linked through a 1,3-bis(methylene)benzene spacer. The **1·4PF$_6$–3·4PF$_6$** salts can be chemisorbed directly on polycrystalline silicon surfaces, whereas the incorporation of a propargyloxy moiety in **4·4PF$_6$** allows its covalent immobilization by copper(I)-catalyzed azide-alkyne cycloaddition (CuAAC).

The synthesis of **1·4PF$_6$–4·4PF$_6$** salts is presented in Scheme 1. Compounds **5** and **2·4PF$_6$** were prepared following protocols previously described in the literature [25,43] (see Supporting Information). On the other hand, the bipyridinium salts **1·4PF$_6$** and **3·4PF$_6$** were obtained by reaction of **5** with the corresponding alkyl halide, iodomethane or hexadecylbromide, obtaining 87% and 85% of yield, respectively, after anion exchange with NH$_4$PF$_6$. For **4·4PF$_6$**, microwave (MW) radiation was used to perform the reaction between the N-methyl-4,4'-bipyridinium iodide and 1,3-dibromomethyl-5-propargyloxy benzene to obtain the corresponding hexafluorophosphate salt with 81% of yield, after anion exchange with NH$_4$PF$_6$ [44].

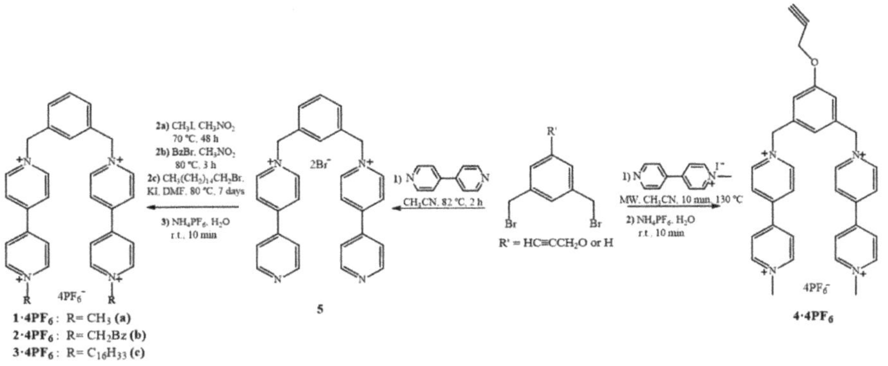

Scheme 1. Synthesis of **5** and bipyridinium salts **1·4PF$_6$**, **2·4PF$_6$**, **3·4PF$_6$** and **4·4PF$_6$**.

The bipyridinium salts **1·4PF$_6$**–**4·4PF$_6$** were characterized by ^{1}H and ^{13}C NMR spectroscopy, MALDI-TOF or HR-ESI mass spectrometry and Infrared (FT-IR) spectroscopy (see Supporting Information, Figures S1–S21).

*3.2. Characterization of Neurotransmitters Complexation with **1·4PF$_6$**–**4·4PF$_6$** in Solution Using Ultraviolet-Visible Absorption and Fluorescence Spectroscopies*

Four π-donor neurotransmitters (**D**, **S**, **A** and **NA**) were selected in this work, to be encapsulated on Poly-Surfs and Poly-Si μPs. This π-donor nature favors the interaction with the π-acceptor bipyridinium salts used as hosts in the non-covalent and covalent functionalization of the polysilicon substrates. The complexation between the neurotransmitters and the π-acceptor hosts (**1·4PF$_6$**–**4·4PF$_6$**) was initially followed by ultraviolet-visible (UV-Vis) absorption spectroscopy in solution. Therefore, the appearance of the corresponding visible charge-transfer (CT) band upon mixing either of **1·4PF$_6$**–**4·4PF$_6$** in DMSO with either **D**, **S**, **A** or **NA** in deionized H$_2$O, indicated the formation of the π-acceptor/π-donor complexes. The use of the mixture DMSO: H$_2$O (4:1) responds to the insolubility of the π-acceptor bipyridinium salts in aqueous solutions. To the naked eye, the complex formation was also evidenced by a solution color change from pale yellow to pink. Figure 2 shows the UV-Vis absorption spectra for the association of the tetracationic hosts **1·4PF$_6$**, **2·4PF$_6$**, **3·4PF$_6$** or **4·4PF$_6$** with **D**, **S**, **A** and **NA** (Figure 2a–d, respectively). For all cases, the characteristic CT bands were observed in a range between 400–600 nm, as it has been reported for similar structures [20]. In this UV-Vis region none of the compounds have an absorbance band (see Supporting Information Figure S22). Furthermore, the results show that **1·4PF$_6$**–**3·4PF$_6$** present higher incorporation of **S**, whereas **4·4PF$_6$** presents a higher interaction with **A**.

Fluorescence spectroscopy was also used to monitor the incorporation of the neurotransmitters in solution. Due to the similar response observed for **1·4PF$_6$**–**3·4PF$_6$** with the neurotransmitters by UV-Vis studies, the fluorescence emission studies were performed using only **1·4PF$_6$** and **4·4PF$_6$**, which have similar structures, and will allow the comparison of the non-covalent and covalent functionalization of the Poly-Surfs. The fluorescence spectra of the neurotransmitters and **1·4PF$_6$** and **4·4PF$_6$**, respectively, in DMSO: H$_2$O (4:1) solution depicted that the bipyridinium salts are not fluorescent (see Supporting Information Figure S23a), whereas all catecholamine-based neurotransmitters (**D**, **A** and **NA**) presented an emission maximum peak at 315 nm, the indolamine-based neurotransmitter (**S**) presented an emission maximum peak at 338 nm (see Supporting Information Figure S23a). Once the neurotransmitters were mixed with either **1·4PF$_6$** and **4·4PF$_6$**, a decrease in their fluorescence intensity was observed, suggesting that the formation of the complex induced fluorescence emission quenching (see Supporting Information Figure S23b,c). All fluorescence spectra were collected at the maximum excitation wavelengths (see Supporting Information, Figure S22).

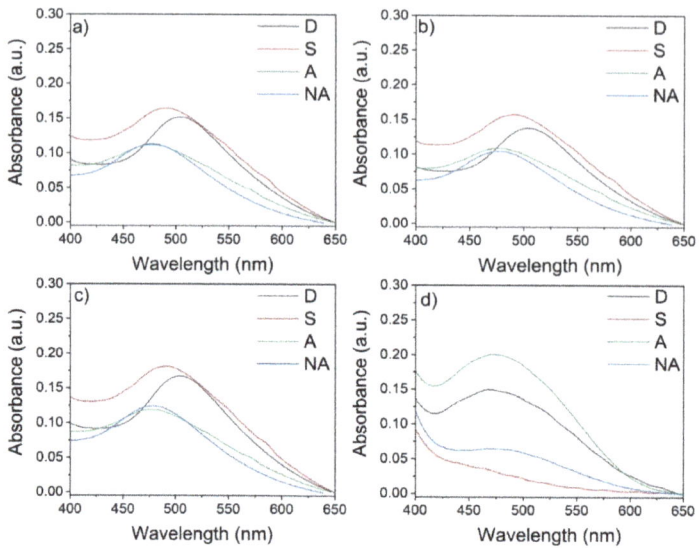

Figure 2. UV-Vis absorption spectra of a mixture of **D**, **S**, **A** or **NA** with: (**a**) **1·4PF$_6$**, (**b**) **2·4PF$_6$**, (**c**) **3·4PF$_6$** and (**d**) **4·4PF$_6$** in 2.5 mL of DMSO:H$_2$O (4:1). The spectra show the corresponding charge-transfer absorption band.

3.3. Functionalization and Characterization of Polysilicon Surfaces and Microparticles with 1·4PF$_6$–4·4PF$_6$ and Neurotransmitter Incorporation

Poly-Surfs and Poly-Si µPs, which are robust and biocompatible materials, were selected to be functionalized with **1·4PF$_6$–3·4PF$_6$** and **4·4PF$_6$** [14,15]. Hence, functionalized polysilicon substrates were explored as carriers for the encapsulation of neurotransmitters (**D**, **S**, **A** or **NA**). The fabrication process of both polysilicon substrates was performed following the protocols previously reported [12,46]. Briefly, a four-inch p-type silicon wafer is used as a starting substrate (Figure 3a). The fabrication process is based in the combination of a 500 nm-thick polysilicon device layer deposited by chemical vapor deposition (CVD) on a 1 µm thermal grown silicon oxide layer that acts as a sacrificial layer (Figure 3b,c). Then, 1.2 µm of photoresist was spun on the polysilicon layer (Figure 3d), to subsequently define the lateral dimensions of the device by a photolithographic step (Figure 3e) followed by a vertical polysilicon dry etching (Figure 3f). Afterwards, the photoresist was removed by plasma etching (Figure 3g). An array of 3 × 3 µm separated 3 µm was obtained (Poly-Surfs). To obtain the Poly-Si µPs, they were released from the array by the etching of the silicon oxide sacrificial layer in vapors of hydrofluoric acid (HF) (Figure 3h). Finally, the released microparticles were suspended in ethanol by using an ultrasonic bath and collected by 5 µm filter rating. Three medium changes are made to the suspended particles by centrifugation to ensure removal of possible traces of HF.

Therefore, the Poly-Surfs used have an area of approximately 1 cm^2 and present a pattern of polysilicon microparticles with lateral dimensions 3 × 3 µm^2 and 0.5 µm thickness on the thermal silicon oxide layer (Figure 4a–c). Moreover, the bipyridinium salts **1·4PF$_6$** and **4·4PF$_6$** were also immobilized on suspended microparticles of 3 × 3 µm^2 and 0.5 µm thickness (Figure 4d–f). Particle size distribution of the Poly-Surfs and Poly-Si µPs suspended in solution were performed, analyzing scanning electron microscope (SEM) and optical microscope images, respectively. The statistics particle size histogram showed an average length of 3.24 ± 0.07 µm for the Poly-Surfs and 3.34 ± 0.11 µm for the Poly-Si µPs (Figure S24). The deviation of each measurement confirmed the high reproducibility of the microparticles achieved using the microfabrication techniques. These dimensions were chosen due to the demonstrated internalization of microparticles with this size into cells and their low toxicity [15].

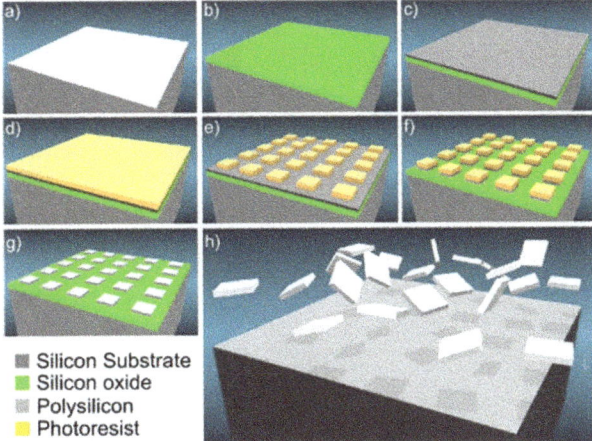

Figure 3. Fabrication of the polysilicon substrates. (**a**) Silicon wafer starting substrate. (**b**) Thermal growing of a 1 μm-thick silicon oxide (sacrificial layer). (**c**) Deposition of a 500 nm-thick CVD polysilicon layer (structural layer). (**d**) 1.2 μm-thick photoresist layer deposition. (**e**) Photolithographic step to define lateral dimensions. (**f**) Vertical dry etching of the polysilicon layer. (**g**) Removing of the photoresist layer to obtain the Poly-Surfs. (**h**) Etching of the sacrificial layer in HF vapors and release of Poly-Si μPs.

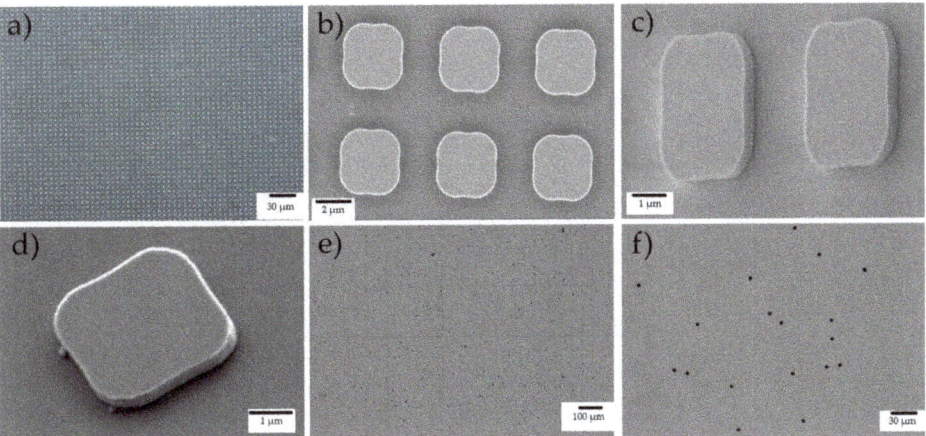

Figure 4. Images of Poly-Surfs with patterned Poly-Si μPs with lateral dimensions 3×3 μm^2 and 0.5 μm thickness on a thermal silicon oxide layer: (**a**) Optical microscope image at scale bar of 30 μm); (**b**,**c**) Scanning electron microscope (SEM) images at scale bars of 2 and 1 μm. Images of etched and suspended Poly-Si μPs: (**d**) SEM image of a single Poly-Si μP; (**e**,**f**) Optical microscope images at scale bar of 100 and 30 μm, respectively.

The functionalization was always first attempted using the Poly-Surfs and the synthetic methodology was then adapted to the Poly-Si μPs' functionalization. Since single-microparticle surface characterization based on common laboratory techniques together with the shape of the Poly-Si μPs is still challenging, the use of the polysilicon surfaces has facilitated the final microparticle surface functionalization and characterization.

Scheme 2 presents the two different approaches used for the immobilization of the host molecules on the Poly-Surfs, the non-covalent with **1·4PF$_6$–3·4PF$_6$** and the covalent with **4·4PF$_6$**. On both strategies, the first step consisted on cleaning and activating the polycrystalline silicon substrates using piranha solution and basic piranha solution. Then, the Poly-Surfs were functionalized by immersing the substrates into a DMSO solution of either **1·4PF$_6$–3·4PF$_6$**. For the covalent immobilization of **4·4PF$_6$**, first an azide-terminated monolayer was prepared using 11-azidoundecyltrimethoxysilane (N$_3$-silane) followed by the azide-alkyne cycloaddition between the azido-functionalized surface and the alkyne moiety of **4·4PF$_6$**. Finally, functionalized substrates with the corresponding bipyridinium salts (**1·4PF$_6$–4·4PF$_6$**) were immersed in an aqueous solution of either **D, S, A** or **NA** to be encapsulated. Additionally, control experiments were made by the immersion of activated Poly-Surfs in a solution of each neurotransmitter (**D, S, A** or **NA**).

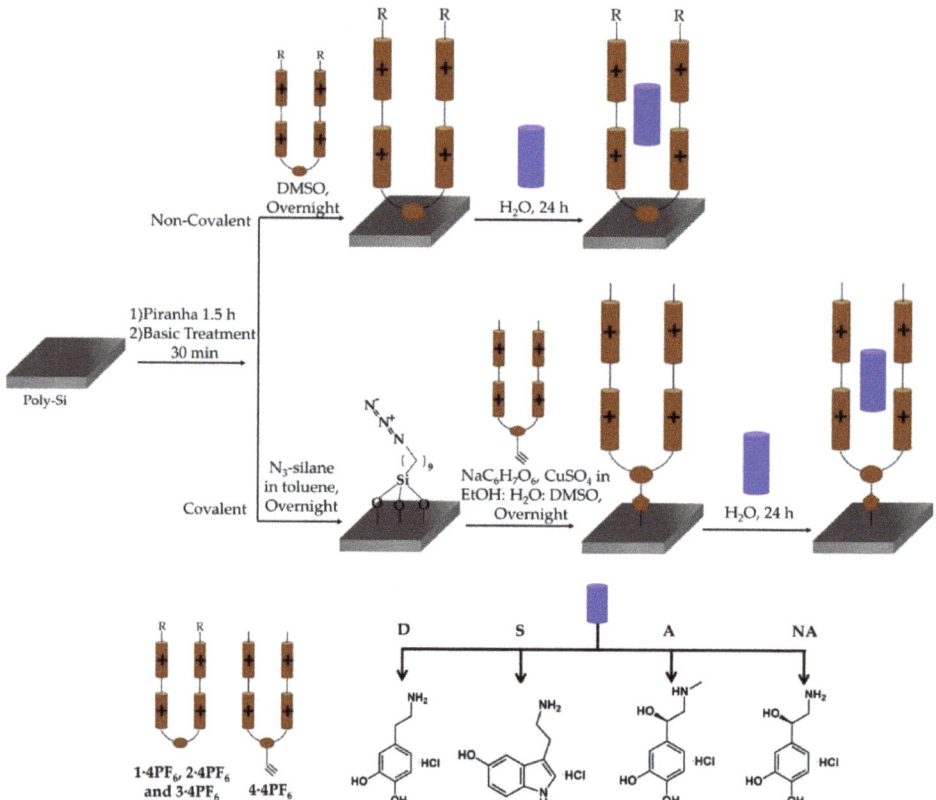

Scheme 2. Functionalization of polysilicon surfaces (Poly-Surfs) and microparticles (Poly-Si μPs) with bipyridinium salts **1·4PF$_6$–4·4PF$_6$** and the subsequent incorporation of **D, S, A** or **NA**. R = CH$_3$ (**1·4PF$_6$**); CH$_2$Bz (**2·4PF$_6$**); C$_{16}$H$_{33}$ (**3·4PF$_6$**).

The functionalization of the Poly-Surfs and the incorporation of the neurotransmitters were characterized by contact angle (θ) measurements, and the values obtained in all functionalization steps are shown in Table 1. The initial polysilicon surfaces exhibit a water contact angle of 44° ± 3. After cleaning and activation steps, a decrease in the contact angle values was observed, obtaining values of 16° ± 2 and 10° ± 1, respectively, and confirming the high hydrophobicity of the surfaces. Functionalized polysilicon surfaces with **1·4PF$_6$–3·4PF$_6$** showed an increase in the contact angle values between θ = 57°–89° ± 1, due to the hydrophobic character of the bipyridinium salts (see Table 1). Moreover, the surface functionalized with **3·4PF$_6$** presented a higher contact angle, due to the longer alkyl chain of 16 carbons, than the rest of the immobilized bipyridinium salts. These results suggest that the polysilicon surfaces were successfully functionalized, and also indicates that the part of the molecule which is facing outwards to the polysilicon surface is the aliphatic moiety, while the polar head is adsorbed onto the surface.

Table 1. Contact angles measurements with the corresponding standard deviation of polysilicon surfaces functionalized with **1·4PF$_6$–4·4PF$_6$**, and subsequent incorporation of neurotransmitters **D**, **S**, **A** and **NA**, and control experiments.

Average Contact Angles (θ) ± Standard Deviation (SD) (°)									
Polysilicon Surfaces							44 ± 3		
After Piranha							16 ± 2		
After Basic Treatment							10 ± 1		
1·4PF$_6$		**2·4PF$_6$**		**3·4PF$_6$**		**4·4PF$_6$**		Controls	
Surface	θ ± SD	Surface	θ ± SD	Surface	θ ± SD	Surface	θ ± SD	Surface	θ ± SD
1·4PF$_6$	57 ± 1	2·4PF$_6$	66 ± 1	3·4PF$_6$	89 ± 1	4·4PF$_6$	55 ± 4	-	
1·4PF$_6$:D	48 ± 1	2·4PF$_6$:D	57 ± 1	3·4PF$_6$:D	73 ± 2	4·4PF$_6$:D	44 ± 3	D	31 ± 3
1·4PF$_6$:S	44 ± 1	2·4PF$_6$:S	55 ± 1	3·4PF$_6$:S	69 ± 2	4·4PF$_6$:S	45 ± 2	S	32 ± 1
1·4PF$_6$:A	40 ± 1	2·4PF$_6$:A	50 ± 2	3·4PF$_6$:A	70 ± 1	4·4PF$_6$:A	48 ± 2	A	30 ± 1
1·4PF$_6$:NA	43 ± 1	2·4PF$_6$:NA	52 ± 2	3·4PF$_6$:NA	66 ± 1	4·4PF$_6$:NA	43 ± 1	NA	30 ± 3

N$_3$-SAM = 78 ± 1.

On the other hand, for the covalent approach, the azido-functionalization presented an hydrophobic contact angle with a value of 78° ± 1, typical for terminal azide-monolayers [47]. After the 1,3-dipolar cycloaddition reaction, the value decreased to 55° ± 4, which is comparable to the value obtained for **1·4PF$_6$**, due to the similarities in their structure, suggesting the formation of the **4·4PF$_6$** layer [48]. After the incorporation of either of the four different water-soluble neurotransmitters (**D**, **S**, **A** or **NA**) on the functionalized polysilicon surfaces, the contact angle values decrease noticeably, as shown in Table 1, indicating the presence of the water-soluble π-electron rich neurotransmitters. This result denotes that the π-donor compounds were incorporated on the polysilicon surfaces through an aromatic π-acceptor/π-donor complex. For the control experiments, an increase in the contact angle values was observed compared to the activation step, suggesting the adsorption of the neurotransmitters onto the activated surfaces. However, the contact angles values were lower than the ones obtained when the bipyridinium salts were immobilized, indicating the successful complex formation [49].

Polysilicon microparticles (3 × 3 µm^2 and 0.5 µm thickness) were then functionalized in suspension with either **1·4PF$_6$** or **4·4PF$_6$**, both having the same peripheral ending group, in order two compare both strategies of functionalization (non-covalent and covalent). The functionalization protocols followed for these substrates were similar to the ones optimized for the functionalization of the Poly-Surfs (Scheme 2). The π-donor neurotransmitter **A** was then selected for its encapsulation on the Poly-Si µPs functionalized with **1·4PF$_6$** or **4·4PF$_6$**.

High-performance liquid chromatography coupled to a fluorescence detector (HPLC-FLD) was used along the experiments with microparticles for the quantification of **A** that is incorporated in them, using excitation and emission wavelengths of 280 and 315 nm, respectively. Therefore, to determine the amount of **A** that can be encapsulated in the microparticles functionalized with either **1·4PF$_6$** or **4·4PF$_6$**, a 2 mM solution of **A** was first prepared (**A$_{in}$** or initial solution). Then, the Poly-Si µPs functionalized with **1·4PF$_6$** or **4·4PF$_6$** were immersed in the **A$_{in}$** solution for 24 h. After this time, microparticles were sedimented by centrifugation and the supernatant was collected (**A$_{fin}$** or final solution). Before **A$_{in}$** and **A$_{fin}$** solutions were injected in the HPLC, a dilution (1:10) was necessary in order to avoid the saturation of the fluorescence detector. Hence, the concentrations of the initial and final solutions were obtained by means of a calibration curve of **A** in the range of 0.18–7.21×10^{-4} mM in deionized H_2O (see Supporting Information, Figures S25 and S26 and Table S1), and the amount of **A** incorporated into the functionalized microparticles was determined by difference. Moreover, in order to estimate the average **A** encapsulated per microparticle, the number of microparticles corresponding to each suspension was also determined by optical microscopy, using a Neubauer chamber (see experimental details, Figure 4e and Equation S1).

The results show that the Poly-Si µPs functionalized with **4·4PF$_6$** can incorporate almost two times more **A** per microparticle (7.8×10^{-8} µmol/particle) than those functionalized with **1·4PF$_6$** (4.3×10^{-8} µmol/particle) (see Supporting Information Table S2). This trend was also observed in the UV-Vis solution experiments, showing that the structural difference between both molecules may have an influence on the host–guest complex formation.

3.4. Release Studies from A Encapsulated in Microparticles

The release of **A** from the functionalized Poly-Si µPs, with **1·4PF$_6$** or **4·4PF$_6$**, was carried out using ascorbic acid (Vitamin C) as the release trigger. Ascorbic acid is a natural compound present in cells, and more importantly, capable of reducing bipyridinium salts, and hence, it may disassemble the supramolecular complex formed by **4·4PF$_6$** and **A**, releasing the encapsulated material [50]. To this end, the dissociation of the **4·4PF$_6$:A** complex was first studied by UV-Vis absorption spectroscopy in solution (see Supporting Information Figure S27). Upon addition of ascorbic acid in a ratio 2:1 (ascorbic: **4·4PF$_6$**), the color of the solution changed from pink to blue, suggesting the reduction in the viologen moieties of **4·4PF$_6$** to their radical cation. In this regard, the UV-Vis spectrum shows the disappearance of the charge-transfer band and the appearance of the bands corresponding to the bipyridinium radical cation at 400 and 600 nm, suggesting the disassembly of the complex in presence of the triggering agent (see Supporting Information Figure S27) [51]. Moreover, the broad band from 250 to 350 nm could be attributed to **A** released (279 nm), the presence of dehydroascorbic acid (300 nm), which is the result of the oxidation of the ascorbic acid, and the excess of the triggering agent used (265 nm) [52].

HPLC coupled to a UV-Vis absorption spectroscopy detector (HPLC-UV-Vis) was also used to study the encapsulation of **A** through the formation of π-acceptor/π-donor complexes (**1·4PF$_6$:A** or **4·4PF$_6$:A**), as well as their disassembly under chromatographic conditions. For that, 2 mM solutions of either **A**, **1·4PF$_6$**, **4·4PF$_6$**, **1·4PF$_6$:A** and **4·4PF$_6$:A** (2 mM: each) were analyzed separately by monitoring the absorption at 479 nm, corresponding to the wavelength of the charge-transfer band of the complex. Chromatograms of either **A, 1·4PF$_6$** or **4·4PF$_6$** show no peaks (besides the solvent front around 1.5–2 min) (see Supporting Information Figure S28a,b,e). However, when analyzing the chromatograms of the complexes (**1·4PF$_6$:A** and **4·4PF$_6$:A**) (Figure S28c and Figure S28f, respectively) new peaks can be observed at retention times of 7.25 and 7.5 min, respectively. In addition, when extracting the corresponding absorption spectra of the samples at these retention times, the absorption spectra clearly show the charge-transfer band (see Supporting Information, Figure S29c,g). These results confirm the successful formation of the complex and its stability under the chromatographic conditions, while the longer retention times (>7 min) as compared to those of the compounds, show the hydrophobic nature of the π-acceptor/π-donor complexes as compared to the compounds separately. Furthermore, once the trigger agent was added to the complexes **1·4PF$_6$:A** and **4·4PF$_6$:A**, the signal corresponding to the complexes at retention time between 7 and 8 min disappeared, confirming the disassembly of the complex upon the reduction in the bipyridinium moiety (see Supporting Information Figure S28d,g). Likewise, the absorption spectra extracted from those chromatograms at the same retention times do not show the charge-transfer absorption band (between 400–600 nm) (see Supporting Information, Figure S29d,h).

To assess if **A** could be released from the Poly-Si µPs functionalized with the complexes **1·4PF$_6$:A** or **4·4PF$_6$:A**, upon an external stimulus, they were incubated in an aqueous solution of ascorbic acid. In order to calculate the amount of **A** released from the functionalized Poly-Si µPs, they were centrifuged and the supernatant was kept (release solution- T1). Moreover, to ensure the maximum amount of **A** released, a second cycle of incubation with ascorbic acid was carried out, obtaining a second release solution (T2). The amount of **A** in the release solutions (T1 and T2) was then analyzed by HPLC coupled to a fluorescence detector set (λ_{exc} = 280 nm and λ_{em} = 315 nm). Since **A** was the only fluorescent compound in the mixture, the areas under the curve (AUC) of the fluorescent peaks at retention time of 2.5 min were measured and the amount of released **A** was obtained by using the calibration curve (see Supporting Information: Figure S25, Figure S30 and Table S3). Particles functionalized with **1·4PF$_6$** can release **A** in the presence of ascorbic acid up to 5.0×10^{-9} µmol/particle, while those functionalized with **4·4PF$_6$** can release up to 4.7×10^{-9} µmol/particle (see Supporting Information Table S4). However, in global a, higher release of **A** was observed for microparticles functionalized with **1·4PF$_6$** (9% of **A** encapsulated) than those functionalized with **4·4PF$_6$** (5% of **A** encapsulated), indicating that, with the covalent approach, a higher amount of the incorporation and lower release of **A** can be assessed (see Supporting Information Table S4).

Finally, in order to ensure that the presence of the ascorbic acid did not affect the physicochemical properties of **A** in the mixture during the release experiments, a stability study was performed. For this purpose, a mixture of **A** and ascorbic acid (1:2 molar ratio) was analyzed every 10 min, for a total of 55 min (the overall time involved in the release experiment) by HPLC-FLD. For all the experiments, the area of the peaks corresponding to **A**, at retention time of 2.5 min, was measured and the concentration of **A** was estimated using the previous calibration curve (see Supporting Information Figure S25). This experiment showed that the concentration of **A** was maintained for at least 55 min, corroborating the stability of **A** during the release experiments (see Supporting Information Figure S31).

3.5. Cytotoxicity and Genotoxicity Assay of 1·4PF$_6$

The non-covalent attachment of **1·4PF$_6$** to the Poly-Si µPs could imply some possible desorption of the compound along time and therefore its toxicity was necessary studied using three different cell lines (3T3/NIH, HepG2 and Caco-2). The cells were exposed to a range of concentrations of compound **1·4PF$_6$** for 24 h. After exposure, the viability of the cell culture was performed using the MTT Assay, and the percentage of viable cells is shown in the Supporting Information (Tables S5–S7). Moreover, IC$_{50}$ values were calculated for the three different cell lines and are shown in the Supporting Information (Table S8). As can be seen, the IC$_{50}$ values (above 122 µM) found for **1·4PF$_6$** suggested very low toxicity in the three cells line used (3T3/NIH, HepG2 and Caco-2), making this compound suitable for biological applications. Furthermore, to evaluate the genotoxicity of **1·4PF$_6$** in the three cell lines (3T3/NIH, HepG2 and Caco-2), the Single-Cell Gel Electrophoresis, also known as Comet Assay, was used according to guidelines [53]. For this analysis, cell viability values higher than 70% are required, and a genotoxic effect is evaluated considering the percentage of tail intensity, which refers to the DNA fragmentation. For instance, tail intensity values higher than 10% are considered genotoxic. As a positive control, the alkylating-agent methyl methanesulfonate (MMS 400 mM) was used. Despite the previously reported high toxicity of viologens, mainly methyl viologen for their use as non-selective herbicide [54], the results showed that **1·4PF$_6$** did not promote a significant formation of DNA fragments within the studied concentrations and cell lines tested. This means that below the IC$_{50}$ values no genotoxicity was observed, confirming the capabilities of these gemini-type amphiphilic bipyridinium salts as promising agents for drug encapsulation and further drug release.

4. Conclusions

In conclusion, we present here a versatile supramolecular approach exploiting π-acceptor/π-donor interactions applied to the encapsulation of π-donor neurotransmitters using π-acceptor aromatic bipyridinium salts functionalized silicon-based materials. With this aim, four different bipyridinium hosts (**1·4PF$_6$**–**4·4PF$_6$**) were synthesized and characterized to incorporate four neurotransmitters (**D**, **S**, **A** and **NA**). The studies in solution using UV-Vis absorption spectroscopy, fluorescence emission spectroscopy and HPLC demonstrated the ability of bipyridinium hosts to form stable supramolecular π-acceptor/π-donor complexes with **D**, **S**, **A** and **NA**. Moreover, **1·4PF$_6$**–**3·4PF$_6$** presented a higher incorporation of **S**, whereas **A** was selectively incorporated by **4·4PF$_6$**. After the solution studies, the immobilization of the **1·4PF$_6$**–**4·4PF$_6$** bipyridinium hosts and incorporation of the neurotransmitters on polysilicon surfaces were accomplished, corroborating each step by contact angle measurements. For the functionalization of polysilicon microparticles, the bipyridinium **1·4PF$_6$** and **4·4PF$_6$** and neurotransmitter **A** were selected. The quantification of **A** encapsulated on the microparticles was assessed by HPLC. Functionalized **4·4PF$_6$** microparticles presented higher encapsulation of **A** than those functionalized with **1·4PF$_6$**, being 7.77×10^{-8} and 4.28×10^{-8} µmol/particle, respectively. Moreover, the release studies in the presence of ascorbic acid indicated similar values of **A** released per particle for **1·4PF$_6$** and **4·4PF$_6$**, being 5.0×10^{-9} and 4.7×10^{-9} µmol/particles, respectively. However, with the non-covalent functionalization of microparticles a higher release of the **A** encapsulated was obtained. Finally, cytotoxicity assays of **1·4PF$_6$** indicated that this bipyridinium host was neither cytotoxic or genotoxic to the cell lines studied 3T3/NIH, HepG2 and Caco-2 at the maximum concentration tested of 500 µg/mL, and therefore a possible desorption of the compound over time from the surfaces will not affect the biocompatibility of the system.

Supplementary Materials: The following are available online at http://www.mdpi.com/1999-4923/12/8/724/s1, Figures S1–S21: Synthesis of **2·4PF$_6$** and **5**, and characterization of **1·4PF$_6$**–**4·4PF$_6$** and **5**, Figure S22: UV-Vis absorption spectra of **1·4PF$_6$**, **4·4PF$_6$**, **D**, **S**, **A** and **NA**, Figure S23: Fluorescence spectra of **1·4PF$_6$**, **4·4PF$_6$**, **D**, **S**, **A** and **NA** and their corresponding complexes, Figure S24: Size distribution study of microparticles, Figure S25: Calibration curve of **A** by HPLC, Equation S(1): Protocol for particles counting using a Neubauer chamber, Figure S26: HPLC-Fluorescence chromatograms of initial and final solutions of **A**, Table S1: Values of retention time (RT) and Area under the curve (AUC) extracted from the chromatograms at Figure S26, Table S2: Quantification of **A** encapsulated in **1·4PF$_6$** and **4·4PF$_6$** functionalized microparticles, Figure S27: UV-Vis solution studies of complex formation (**4·4PF$_6$:A**) and disassembly using ascorbic acid, Figure S28: HPLC solution studies of complex formation (**4·4PF$_6$:A**) and disassembly using ascorbic acid, Figure S29: HPLC-UV-Vis absorption spectra of complex formation (**1·4PF$_6$:A** and **4·4PF$_6$:A**) and disassembly, Figure S30: HPLC-Fluorescence chromatograms of release solutions (T1 and T2) of **A** after adding ascorbic acid to the functionalized microparticles, Table S3: Values of retention time (RT) and Area under the curve (AUC) extracted from the chromatograms at Figure S30, Table S4: Quantification of **A** released in **1·4PF$_6$** and **4·4PF$_6$** functionalized microparticles by using ascorbic acid, Figure S31: Stability studies of **A** in presence of ascorbic acid, Table S5: Results obtained for cell viability and genotoxicity results for **1·4PF$_6$** in cell line 3T3/NIH, Table S6: Results obtained for cell viability and genotoxicity results for **1·4PF$_6$** in cell line HepG2, Table S7: Results obtained for cell viability and genotoxicity results for **1·4PF$_6$** in cell line Caco-2 and Table S8: Values of the IC$_{50}$ determined for the compound **1·4PF$_6$** tested in the three different cell lines (3T3/NIH, HepG2 and Caco-2).

Author Contributions: Conceptualization, A.G.-C., A.G. and L.P.-G.; silicon-based materials fabrication, M.D. and J.A.P.; experimental part, S.G. and M.E.A.-R.; HPLC experiments, S.G. and D.L.; cytotoxicity and genotoxicity assays, D.R.-L. and J.d.L.; resources, A.G.-C. and L.P.G.; writing—review and editing, S.G., M.E.A.-R, D.L., A.G.-C. and L.P.-G.; supervision, A.G.-C., A.G. and L.P.-G.; funding acquisition, A.G.-C. and L.P.-G. All authors have read and agreed to the published version of the manuscript.

Funding: This research was funded by EU ERDF (FEDER) funds and the Spanish Government grant TEC2017-85059-C3-1-1-R and -2-R and MAT2016-77852-C2-1-R (AEI/FEDER, UE).

Acknowledgments: The project thanks the support from Generalitat de Catalunya (SGR-1277). S.G. thanks MINECO for a predoctoral grant (FPI). A.G.-C. acknowledges financial support from the Spanish Ministry of Economy and Competitiveness, through the "Severo Ochoa" Programme for Centers of Excellence in R&D (SEV-2015-0496) and the Ministry of Science and Innovation for a Ramon y Cajal contract (RYC-2017-22910).

Conflicts of Interest: The authors declare no conflict of interest.

References

1. Bah, M.G.; Bilal, H.M.; Wang, J. Fabrication and application of complex microcapsules: A review. *Soft Matter* **2020**, *16*, 570–590. [CrossRef] [PubMed]
2. Panwar, N.; Soehartono, A.M.; Chan, K.K.; Zeng, S.; Xu, G.; Qu, J.; Coquet, P.; Yong, K.T.; Chen, X. Nanocarbons for Biology and Medicine: Sensing, Imaging, and Drug Delivery. *Chem. Rev.* **2019**, *119*, 9559–9656. [CrossRef] [PubMed]
3. Manzano, M.; Vallet-Regí, M. Mesoporous Silica Nanoparticles for Drug Delivery. *Adv. Funct. Mater.* **2020**, *30*, 3–5. [CrossRef]

4. Shalek, A.K.; Robinson, J.T.; Karp, E.S.; Lee, J.S.; Ahn, D.R.; Yoon, M.H.; Sutton, A.; Jorgolli, M.; Gertner, R.S.; Gujral, T.S.; et al. Vertical silicon nanowires as a universal platform for delivering biomolecules into living cells. *Proc. Natl. Acad. Sci. USA* **2010**, *107*, 1870–1875. [CrossRef]
5. Siqueira, J.R.; Caseli, L.; Crespilho, F.N.; Zucolotto, V.; Oliveira, O.N. Immobilization of biomolecules on nanostructured films for biosensing. *Biosens. Bioelectron.* **2010**, *25*, 1254–1263. [CrossRef]
6. Cheng, F.; Shang, J.; Ratner, D.M. A versatile method for functionalizing surfaces with bioactive glycans. *Bioconjug. Chem.* **2011**, *22*, 50–57. [CrossRef]
7. Singh, M.; Kaur, N.; Comini, E. The role of self-assembled monolayers in electronic devices. *J. Mater. Chem. C* **2020**, *8*, 3938–3955. [CrossRef]
8. Zhang, L.; Wang, Z.; Das, J.; Labib, M.; Ahmed, S.; Sargent, E.H.; Kelley, S.O. Potential-Responsive Surfaces for Manipulation of Cell Adhesion, Release, and Differentiation. *Angew. Chem. Int. Ed.* **2019**, *58*, 14519–14523. [CrossRef]
9. Qiu, M.; Singh, A.; Wang, D.; Qu, J.; Swihart, M.; Zhang, H.; Prasad, P.N. Biocompatible and biodegradable inorganic nanostructures for nanomedicine: Silicon and black phosphorus. *Nano Today* **2019**, *25*, 135–155. [CrossRef]
10. Koch, B.; Rubino, I.; Quan, F.S.; Yoo, B.; Choi, H.J. Microfabrication for drug delivery. *Materials* **2016**, *9*, 646. [CrossRef] [PubMed]
11. Xu, Y.; Hu, X.; Kundu, S.; Nag, A.; Afsarimanesh, N.; Sapra, S.; Mukhopadhyay, S.C.; Han, T. Silicon-Based Sensors for Biomedical Applications: A Review. *Sensors* **2019**, *19*, 2908. [CrossRef] [PubMed]
12. Bruce, G.; Samperi, M.; Amabilino, D.B.; Duch, M.; Plaza, J.A.; Pérez-García, L. Singlet oxygen generation from porphyrin-functionalized hexahedral polysilicon microparticles. *J. Porphyr. Phthalocyanines* **2019**, *23*, 223–233. [CrossRef]
13. Penon, O.; Siapkas, D.; Novo, S.; Durán, S.; Oncins, G.; Errachid, A.; Barrios, L.; Nogués, C.; Duch, M.; Plaza, J.A.; et al. Optimized immobilization of lectins using self-assembled monolayers on polysilicon encoded materials for cell tagging. *Colloids Surf. B Biointerfaces* **2014**, *116*, 104–113. [CrossRef] [PubMed]
14. Penon, O.; Novo, S.; Durán, S.; Ibañez, E.; Nogués, C.; Samitier, J.; Duch, M.; Plaza, J.A.; Pérez-García, L. Efficient biofunctionalization of polysilicon barcodes for adhesion to the zona pellucida of mouse embryos. *Bioconjug. Chem.* **2012**, *23*, 2392–2402. [CrossRef]
15. Fernández-Rosas, E.; Gómez, R.; Ibañez, E.; Barrios, L.; Duch, M.; Esteve, J.; Plaza, J.A.; Nogués, C. Internalization and cytotoxicity analysis of silicon-based microparticles in macrophages and embryos. *Biomed. Microdevices* **2010**, *12*, 371–379. [CrossRef]
16. Patiño, T.; Soriano, J.; Amirthalingam, E.; Durán, S.; González-Campo, A.; Duch, M.; Ibáñez, E.; Barrios, L.; Plaza, J.A.; Pérez-García, L.; et al. Polysilicon-chromium-gold intracellular chips for multi-functional biomedical applications. *Nanoscale* **2016**, *8*, 8773–8783. [CrossRef]
17. Durán, S.; Duch, M.; Gómez-Martínez, R.; Fernández-Regúlez, M.; Agusil, J.P.; Reina, M.; Müller, C.; Paulo, Á.S.; Esteve, J.; Castel, S.; et al. Internalization and viability studies of suspended nanowire silicon chips in hela cells. *Nanomaterials* **2020**, *10*, 893.
18. Li, Z.; Song, N.; Yang, Y.W. Stimuli-Responsive Drug-Delivery Systems Based on Supramolecular Nanovalves. *Matter* **2019**, *1*, 345–368. [CrossRef]
19. Goodnow, T.T.; Reddington, M.V.; Stoddart, J.F.; Kaifer, A.E. Cyclobis(paraquat-p-phenylene): A Novel Synthetic Receptor for Amino Acids with Electron-Rich Aromatic Moieties. *J. Am. Chem. Soc.* **1991**, *113*, 4335–4337. [CrossRef]
20. Bernardo, A.R.; Stoddart, J.F.; Kaifer, A.E. Cyclobis(paraquat-p-phenylene) as a Synthetic Receptor for Electron-Rich Aromatic Compounds: Electrochemical and Spectroscopic Studies of Neurotransmitter Binding. *J. Am. Chem. Soc.* **1992**, *114*, 10624–10631. [CrossRef]
21. Raymo, F.M.; Cejas, M.A. Supramolecular association of dopamine with immobilized fluorescent probes. *Org. Lett.* **2002**, *4*, 3183–3185. [CrossRef] [PubMed]
22. Cejas, M.A.; Raymo, F.M. Fluorescent diazapyrenium films and their response to dopamine. *Langmuir* **2005**, *21*, 5795–5802. [CrossRef] [PubMed]
23. Anelli, P.L.; Ashton, P.R.; Philp, D.; Pietraszkiewicz, M.; Reddington, M.V.; Spencer, N.; Stoddart, J.F.; Vicent, C.; Ballardini, R.; Balzani, V.; et al. Molecular Meccano. 1. [2]Rotaxanes and a [2]Catenane Made to Order. *J. Am. Chem. Soc.* **1992**, *114*, 193–218. [CrossRef]

24. Amabilino, D.B.; Ashton, P.R.; Brown, C.L.; Newton, S.P.; Pietraszkiewicz, M.; Philp, D.; Raymo, F.M.; Reder, A.S.; Rutland, M.T.; Spencer, N.; et al. Molecular Meccano. 2 Self-Assembly of [n] Catenanes. *J. Am. Chem. Soc.* **1995**, *117*, 1271–1293. [CrossRef]
25. Ashton, P.R.; Pérez-García, L.; Stoddart, J.F.; Ballardini, R.; Balzani, V.; Credi, A.; Gandolfi, M.T.; Prodi, L.; Venturi, M.; Menzer, S.; et al. Molecular Meccano. 4. The Self-Assembly of [2] Catenanes Incorporating Photoactive and Electroactive π-Extended Systems. *J. Am. Chem. Soc.* **1995**, *117*, 11171–11197.
26. Jordão, N.; Cruz, H.; Branco, A.; Pina, F.; Branco, L.C. Bis(bipyridinium) Salts as Multicolored Electrochromic Devices. *Chempluschem* **2017**, *82*, 1211–1217. [CrossRef]
27. Clarke, D.E.; Olesińska, M.; Mönch, T.; Schoenaers, B.; Stesmans, A.; Scherman, O.A. Aryl-viologen pentapeptide self-assembled conductive nanofibers. *Chem. Commun.* **2019**, *55*, 7354–7357. [CrossRef]
28. Škorjanc, T.; Shetty, D.; Olson, M.A.; Trabolsi, A. Design strategies and redox-dependent applications of insoluble viologen-based covalent organic polymers. *ACS Appl. Mater. Interfaces* **2019**, *11*, 6705–6716. [CrossRef]
29. Guerrini, L.; Garcia-Ramos, J.V.; Domingo, C.; Sanchez-Cortes, S. Nanosensors based on viologen functionalized silver nanoparticles: Few molecules surface-enhanced Raman spectroscopy detection of polycyclic aromatic hydrocarbons in interparticle hot spots. *Anal. Chem.* **2009**, *81*, 1418–1425. [CrossRef]
30. Sultanova, E.D.; Krasnova, E.G.; Kharlamov, S.V.; Nasybullina, G.R.; Yanilkin, V.V.; Nizameev, I.R.; Kadirov, M.K.; Mukhitova, R.K.; Zakharova, L.Y.; Ziganshina, A.Y.; et al. Thermoresponsive polymer nanoparticles based on viologen cavitands. *Chempluschem* **2015**, *80*, 217–222. [CrossRef]
31. Ryu, J.H.; Lee, J.H.; Han, S.J.; Suh, K. Do Influence of viologen lengths on the response time of the reflective electrochromic display prepared by monodisperse viologen-modified polymeric microspheres. *Colloids Surf. A Physicochem. Eng. Asp.* **2008**, *315*, 31–37. [CrossRef]
32. Liu, A.; Han, S.; Che, H.; Hua, L. Fluorescent hybrid with electron acceptor methylene viologen units inside the pore walls of mesoporous MCM-48 silica. *Langmuir* **2010**, *26*, 3555–3561. [CrossRef] [PubMed]
33. Yamanoi, Y.; Nishihara, H. Assembly of nanosize metallic particles and molecular wires on electrode surfaces. *Chem. Commun.* **2007**, 3983–3989. [CrossRef] [PubMed]
34. Liu, X.; Ne, K.G.; Kang, E.T. Viologen-Functionalized Conductive Surfaces: Physicochemical and Electrochemical Characteristics, and Stability. *Langmuir* **2002**, *18*, 9041–9047. [CrossRef]
35. Sou, K.; Le, D.L.; Sato, H. Nanocapsules for Programmed Neurotransmitter Release: Toward Artificial Extracellular Synaptic Vesicles. *Small* **2019**, *15*, 1–12. [CrossRef]
36. Si, B.; Song, E. Recent advances in the detection of neurotransmitters. *Chemosensors* **2018**, *6*, 1. [CrossRef]
37. Niyonambaza, S.D.; Kumar, P.; Xing, P.; Mathault, J.; De Koninck, P.; Boisselier, E.; Boukadoum, M.; Miled, A. A Review of neurotransmitters sensing methods for neuro-engineering research. *Appl. Sci.* **2019**, *9*, 4719. [CrossRef]
38. Teleanu, D.M.; Chircov, C.; Grumezescu, A.M.; Teleanu, R.I. Neuronanomedicine: An up-to-date overview. *Pharmaceutics* **2019**, *11*, 101. [CrossRef]
39. Le, D.L.; Ferdinandus; Tnee, C.K.; Vo Doan, T.T.; Arai, S.; Suzuki, M.; Sou, K.; Sato, H. Neurotransmitter-Loaded Nanocapsule Triggers On-Demand Muscle Relaxation in Living Organism. *ACS Appl. Mater. Interfaces* **2018**, *10*, 37812–37819. [CrossRef]
40. Ragusa, A.; Priore, P.; Giudetti, A.M.; Ciccarella, G.; Gaballo, A. Neuroprotective investigation of Chitosan nanoparticles for dopamine delivery. *Appl. Sci.* **2018**, *8*, 474. [CrossRef]
41. Lai, C.Y.; Trewyn, B.G.; Jeftinija, D.M.; Jeftinija, K.; Xu, S.; Jeftinija, S.; Lin, V.S.Y. A mesoporous silica nanosphere-based carrier system with chemically removable CdS nanoparticle caps for stimuli-responsive controlled release of neurotransmitters and drug molecules. *J. Am. Chem. Soc.* **2003**, *125*, 4451–4459. [CrossRef] [PubMed]
42. Gattuso, G.; Notti, A.; Pappalardo, S.; Parisi, M.F.; Pisagatti, I.; Patanè, S. Encapsulation of monoamine neurotransmitters and trace amines by amphiphilic anionic calix[5]arene micelles. *New J. Chem.* **2014**, *38*, 5983–5990. [CrossRef]
43. Geuder, W.; Hünig, S.; Suchy, A. Single and double bridged viologenes and intramolecular pimerization of their cation radicals. *Tetrahedron* **1986**, *42*, 1665–1677. [CrossRef]
44. Lamberto, M.; Rastede, E.E.; Decker, J.; Raymo, F.M. Microwave-assisted synthesis of symmetric and asymmetric viologens. *Tetrahedron Lett.* **2010**, *51*, 5618–5620. [CrossRef]

45. He, C.; Li, L.W.; He, W.D.; Jiang, W.X.; Wu, C. "Click" long seesaw-type A~~B~A chains together into huge defect-free hyperbranched polymer chains with uniform subchains. *Macromolecules* **2011**, *44*, 6233–6236. [CrossRef]
46. Gómez-Martínez, R.; Vázquez, P.; Duch, M.; Muriano, A.; Pinacho, D.; Sanvicens, N.; Sánchez-Baeza, F.; Boya, P.; De La Rosa, E.J.; Esteve, J.; et al. Intracellular silicon chips in living cells. *Small* **2010**, *6*, 499–502. [CrossRef]
47. Prakash, S.; Long, T.M.; Selby, J.C.; Moore, J.S.; Shannon, M.A. "Click" modification of silica surfaces and glass microfluidic channels. *Anal. Chem.* **2007**, *79*, 1661–1667. [CrossRef]
48. Tian, F.; Cheng, N.; Nouvel, N.; Geng, J.; Scherman, O.A. Site-selective immobilization of colloids on au substrates via a noncovalent supramolecular "handcuff". *Langmuir* **2010**, *26*, 5323–5328. [CrossRef]
49. Sun, Z.; Xi, L.; Zheng, K.; Zhang, Z.; Baldridge, K.K.; Olson, M.A. Classical and non-classical melatonin receptor agonist-directed micellization of bipyridinium- based supramolecular amphiphiles in water. *Soft Matter* **2020**, *16*, 4788–4799. [CrossRef]
50. Janghel, E.K.; Gupta, V.K.; Rai, M.K.; Rai, J.K. Micro determination of ascorbic acid using methyl viologen. *Talanta* **2007**, *72*, 1013–1016. [CrossRef]
51. Watanabe, T.; Honda, K. Measurement of the extinction coefficient of the methyl viologen cation radical and the efficiency of its formation by semiconductor photocatalysis. *J. Phys. Chem.* **1982**, *86*, 2617–2619. [CrossRef]
52. Bradshaw, M.P.; Prenzler, P.D.; Scollary, G.R. Ascorbic acid-induced browning of (+)-catechin in a model wine system. *J. Agric. Food Chem.* **2001**, *49*, 934–939. [CrossRef] [PubMed]
53. ASTM-E2186. *Standard Guide for Determining DNA Single-Strand Damage in Eukaryotic Cells Using the Comet Assay*; ASTM International: West Conshohocken, PA, USA, 2003; Volume 11, pp. 1–12. Available online: https://www.astm.org/DATABASE.CART/HISTORICAL/E2186-02A.htm (accessed on 25 July 2016).
54. Kui, W.; Guo, D.S.; Zhang, H.Q.; Dong, L.; Zheng, X.L.; Yu, L. Highly effective binding of viologens by p-sulfonatocalixarenes for the treatment of viologen poisoning. *J. Med. Chem.* **2009**, *52*, 6402–6412.

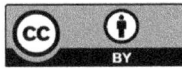

© 2020 by the authors. Licensee MDPI, Basel, Switzerland. This article is an open access article distributed under the terms and conditions of the Creative Commons Attribution (CC BY) license (http://creativecommons.org/licenses/by/4.0/).

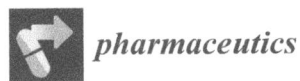

Article

Encapsulating TGF-β1 Inhibitory Peptides P17 and P144 as a Promising Strategy to Facilitate Their Dissolution and to Improve Their Functionalization

Nemany A. N. Hanafy [1,*], Isabel Fabregat [2], Stefano Leporatti [3,*] and Maged El Kemary [1]

1. Nanomedicine Department, Institute of Nanoscience and Nanotechnology, Kafrelsheikh University, Kafrelsheikh 33516, Egypt; elkemary@yahoo.com
2. Bellvitge Biomedical Research Institute (IDIBELL), University of Barcelona (UB) and CIBEREHD, Gran Via de l'Hospitalet, 199, Hospitalet de Llobregat, 08908 Barcelona, Spain; ifabregat@idibell.cat
3. CNR NANOTEC-Istituto di Nanotecnologia, Via Monteroni, 73100 Lecce, Italy
* Correspondence: nemany.hanafy@nano.kfs.edu.eg (N.A.N.H.); stefano.leporatti@nanotec.cnr.it (S.L.)

Received: 24 March 2020; Accepted: 29 April 2020; Published: 2 May 2020

Abstract: Transforming growth factor-beta (TGFβ1) is considered as a master regulator for many intracellular signaling pathways, including proliferation, differentiation and death, both in health and disease. It further represents an oncogenic factor in advanced tumors allowing cancer cells to be more invasive and prone to move into the metastatic process. This finding has received great attention for discovering new therapeutic molecules against the TGFβ1 pathway. Among many TGFβ1 inhibitors, peptides (P17 and P144) were designed to block the TGFβ1 pathway. However, their therapeutic applications have limited use, due to lack of selection for their targets and their possible recognition by the immune system and further due to their potential cytotoxicity on healthy cells. Besides that, P144 is a highly hydrophobic molecule with less dissolution even in organic solution. Here, we aimed to overcome the dissolution of P144, as well as design nano-delivery strategies to protect normal cells, to increase cellular penetration and to raise the targeted therapy of both P17 and P144. Peptides were encapsulated in moieties of polymer hybrid protein. Their assembly was investigated by TEM, microplate spectrum analysis and fluorescence microscopy. SMAD phosphorylation was analyzed by Western blot as a hallmark of their biological efficiency. The results showed that the encapsulation of P17 and P144 might improve their potential therapeutic applications.

Keywords: transforming growth factors; proliferation; polymer hybrid protein

1. Introduction

Transforming growth factor (TGFβ) is a secreted cytokine, having the ability to regulate and control cell proliferation, migration, differentiation and cytoskeleton morphology [1–3]. Apart from this fact, the role of TGFβ in controlling inflammation, wound healing and tissue repair received a lot of interest [4]. However, its function as a tumor promoter at the end stage of cancer development resulted in an impact issue, since it supports cancer growth, activates tumor angiogenesis and inhibits immune responses [5–7]. Among many molecules that were used to inhibit TGFβ signaling pathway, TGFβ inhibitory peptides have obtained great interest due to their efficient role in blocking of TGFβ signaling pathways [8]. Peptide P144, TSLDASIIWAMMQN, is a very hydrophobic peptide obtained from the membrane-proximal ligand-binding domain of b-glycan [9]. This peptide is designed to block TGFβR III extracellular domains preventing cellular interaction between TGF ligand and its receptors [10]. Another soluble peptide is called P17, (KRIWFIPRSSWYERA) [11]. It was produced from a phage library [12]. P17 can block TGF-β1, TGFβ2 and TGFβ3 with relative affinity binding reached 100%, 80% and 30% respectively [13]. The active inhibitory effect of both peptides was characterized in vivo and in vitro for several models of fibrosis and scleroderma [14]. Results have proven the potential therapeutic value for both peptides to block the TGFβ pathway and to prevent the accumulation of collagen fibers [15]. However, there is an urgent needing strategy to improve their dissolution, prevent their aggregation and facilitate their delivery into animal models. P144 was used previously either after it is suspended inside dimethyl sulfoxide (DMSO)-saline [16] or, after its integration into the composition of the lipogel in the presence of 5% DMSO [17]. Both strategies were restricted due to the presence of DMSO [18]. Additionally, both peptides can be distributed into the whole body, with no specific delivery into a certain region. Leading to increase their accumulation inside healthy tissues. Additionally, due to their amino acid structure, they can be recognized in the bloodstream and then can be engulfed by the immune system or can be degraded inside the stomach by a biological enzyme [19]. In the current study, the sonicated P144 and suspended P17 were internalized into the bovine serum albumin matrix through amino–carboxyl interaction. Such attachment is characterized by strong interaction between peptide and protein due to the presence of carboxyl, amino-groups and hydrogen intermolecular interactions.

Additionally, the surface of the protein–peptide complex was further functionalized by folic-acid-attached carboxymethyl cellulose (CMC; Supplementary Scheme S1A). Folic acid is used as a ligand and can bind folate receptors. Additionally, CMC has mucoadhesive properties and allows protein–peptide formulation to adhere and penetrate mucus layers. This strategy provides a novel and concrete reason to strengthen the potential application of peptides as a targeted delivery. The efficiency of encapsulated peptides (P144 and P17) and the pure peptides (with no addition of DMSO or integration into lipogel) were studied by using two different hepatocellular carcinomas (HCC) cell lines: hepatitis B-positive SNU449 cells, [20], that were characterized by a mesenchymal phenotype expression [21] and the human epithelial HCC Hep3B cells [22] with different genetic characterization.

2. Materials and Methods

2.1. Chemicals

The suppliers of the chemicals were as follows. Carboxy methylcellulose (CMC) was purchased from Fluka, Sigma-Aldrich (St. Louis, MO, USA), phosphate-buffered saline (PBS) tablets of pH 7.3 were purchased from Oxoid Limited Basingstoke (Hampshire, England); ethanol from Baker Analyzed, Fisher Scientific, (Landsmeer, The Netherlands); bovine serum albumin (BSA), folic acid (FA), crystal violet, 40,6-diamidino-2-phenylindole dihydrochloride (DAPI), paraformaldehyde, N-ethyl-N0- (3 dimethylaminopropyl)carbodiimide hydrochloride (EDAC), N-hydroxy succinimide (NHS), dimethyl sulfoxide (DMSO) from Sigma-Aldrich (St. Louis, MO, USA).

2.2. Fabrication of Protein–Peptide Mucoadhesive Carriers

A 1 mg amount of sonicated P144 and suspended P17 was mixed into BSA solution (50 µg/50 mL). Then, the mixture will be grafted by carboxymethyl cellulose inside sterilized glass vials for 30 min under rotation by a magnetic stirrer in the presence of EDAC/NHS. The complex was further coated by 5 mL of 50 µg/50 mL protamine and the stirrer was continued into addition for 10 min. Afterward, the mixture was furthermore covered by folic-acid-attached carboxymethyl cellulose and the rotation was completed in an additional 15 min. Un-reacted materials were removed by using a dialysis bag against distilled water for 48 h. The water was changed several times. Then, the final product was lyophilized at a freeze-drying machine while the material was kept at −20 °C until use.

2.3. Characterization of the Protein-Peptides Mucoadhesive Formulation

2.3.1. Transmission Electron Microscopy (TEM)

A 10 µL volume of nanoparticle suspension was deposited on the copper grid and air-dried before measurement. Copper grids sputtered with carbon films were used to support the sample.

High-resolution TEM images of nanoparticles were analyzed by a Hitachi HT 7700 operating (Hitachi, Japan) at 100 kV, coupled with a GATAN camera ORIUS SC600 (Gatan, Inc., Pleasanton, CA, USA)) with a resolution of 7 megapixels. The GATAN camera is controlled by Digital Micrograph (Gatan, Inc., Pleasanton, CA, USA) [23]

2.3.2. UV–Vis Spectroscopy

The absorbance of folic acid and rhodamine was measured by using a multiplate reader at the option of UV Absorbance Spectrophotometer in multiplate wells. A 500 µL mL volume of fabricated nanoparticles was scanned at a range of 300–600 nm [24].

2.3.3. Zeta Potential

The electrophoretic mobility of samples was determined by photon correlation spectroscopy by using a Zeta Nano Sizer (Malvern Instruments, Malvern, UK). All measurements were performed at 25 °C. Five following measurements were taken for analysis; each was run five times with a delay of 5 s after each measurement [25].

2.3.4. ImageJ Analysis and Calculation of the Surface Roughness

The measurements for the light microscopic images (400 µm) were carried out in pixels. Thus, setting up a scale bar for calibration for the calculation of the actual area was not required. Since, in the "Image" option of ImageJ, under Adjust, "size" was selected. Then, the pixel of width and length was adjusted and it is followed by using the "Surface Plot" option in "Analyze". This led to the area measurement of the complete image in pixels.

The measured peaks upon the material surface expressed the status of material that was either roughness or granules, while no peaks were measured in the case of soft materials or those that did not contain any granulated materials [26].

2.4. Cell Culture

Hep3B and SNU449 cells were obtained from the European Collection of Cell Cultures (ECACC). Cell lines were never used in the laboratory for longer than 4 months after receipt or resuscitation. All cells were maintained in DMEM media (Lonza, Basel, Switzerland) supplemented with 10% FBS (Sera Laboratories International Ltd., West Sussex, UK), penicillin (100 U/mL), streptomycin (100 µg/mL), amphotericin (2.5 µg/mL) and L-glutamine (2 mM). They were maintained in a humidified atmosphere at 37 °C and 5% CO_2. Cells were observed under an Olympus IX-70 microscope.

2.4.1. Cellular Uptake

Ten thousand human liver cancer cell lines were seeded upon the surface of a sterilized cover slip that was laid in the bottom of 6 multi-well microplates. After 24 h from their growth, encapsulated peptides and non-encapsulated (50 µg/mL) were added to each well and incubated in a humidified atmosphere of 37 °C, 5% CO_2. SNU449 and Hep3B cell lines were fixed by 4% paraformaldehyde then washed by PBS (phosphate-buffered saline) at pH 7.2. Cells were then stained by DAPI (nuclear stain) for 30 min and washed twice by PBS,7.2. Cellular uptake was analyzed after 24 h by red (TRITC), green (FITC) and blue (DAPI) channels of fluorescence microscopy. After that, images were captured by fluorescence microscopy with a digital camera [27,28].

2.4.2. Proliferation Assay

To evaluate cell proliferation, crystal violet assay was performed at 3, 6, 12, 24, 48 and 72 h [29]. Briefly, 7×10^3 cells/well were seeded in 96-well flat-bottom plates and allowed to grow for 24 h. Encapsulated peptides (P17 and P144) and free capsules were then added at different concentrations (10, 50, 100, 200 µg/mL). After incubation for a certain time, DMEM media was removed and cells were washed using PBS 3 times. Cells were then fixed for 10 min in a solution of buffered formalin (3.7%), and then cells were washed with PBS (pH 7.3) and subsequently stained with a 0.01% crystal violet solution. After removing excess stain, the crystal violet stained cells were dissolved in 1 mL of a 10% sodium dodecyl sulfate solution for 2 h under orbital shaking and the optical density of the extracted dye was read with a spectrophotometer at 590 nm. Optical density measurements give an indication of the relative number of viable cells present at the time of adding dye and this is used to create survival curves. Cell survival at each dose point was expressed as a percentage of the control survival rate.

2.4.3. Western Blot Analysis

Total protein extracts were obtained as described previously [30], separated by SDS/PAGE (12% polyacrylamide gels) and transferred on to PVDF membranes. After blocking with 5% (*w/v*) non-fat milk TBST (Tris-buffered saline solution containing 0.05% (*v/v*) Tween 20), the membranes were incubated overnight with the corresponding antibody in a 0.5% non-fat milk TBST (diluted 1:5000 for β-actin and 1:1000 for all others). After washing and incubating the membrane with an appropriate peroxidase-conjugated antibody (diluted 1:5000) for 1 h at 21 °C, antibody binding was revealed using ECL® (GE-Healthcare). β-actin was used as a loading control.

2.5. Ethical Approval

All experiments were conducted in accordance with US National Institutes of Health Guidelines for the Care and Use of Laboratory Animals and cell line experiments Guide for the Care and Use of Laboratory Animals after being approved by the relevant Ethical Committee and authorized by the Italian and German Ministry of Health. This study was also approved by the Research Ethics Committee of Kafrelsheikh University.

3. Results

3.1. Physical Properties of Peptide P17 and P144

P144 is a very hydrophobic peptide, has a limited dissolution either inside aqueous solution or even in an organic solvent such as DMSO (Figure 1A,B) [10]. This drawback leads to a reduction of its delivery into preclinical studies and minimizes its potential applications. The dissolution of bulk P144 was obtained by using physical sonication for 15 min under high amplitude to prevent microscopic bubbles in solution. After sonication, the bulk of P144 was separated into a colloidal suspension containing small peptide particles (Figure 1C,D). However, these small particles turned into aggregation after their precipitation (Figure 1G). The bulk of P144 is formed by tiny small molecules held together by electrostatic force. These small particles had lost their ionic balance after their separation. For this reason, the separated particles of P144 tend to bind back forming an aggregated state. Contrarily, P17 is very soluble in water, forming a colloidal suspension with good stability [11]. Meanwhile, P17 has a widescreen attachment with three TGFβ isoforms such as TGFβ1, TGFβ2 and TGFβ3.

To investigate their properties with fluorophore conjugation and to follow their cellular uptake, the anti-TGFβ inhibitory peptides (P17 and P144) were labeled by rhodamine (RG6; Figure 1G) [31]. Rhodamine-labeled peptides showed strong absorbance at 550 nm associated with a peak of pure rhodamine [32]. Their interaction is attributed to the amino group of rhodamine and the carboxyl group of peptides. It is noticed that rhodamine-doped peptides have a strengthened second peak localized at 490 nm. This peak emitted green fluorescence with fluorescence microscopy (Figure 1G,H). In addition, sonicated P144 and dissolved P17 were shown as aggregated peptides even after their cellular uptake (Figure 1H).

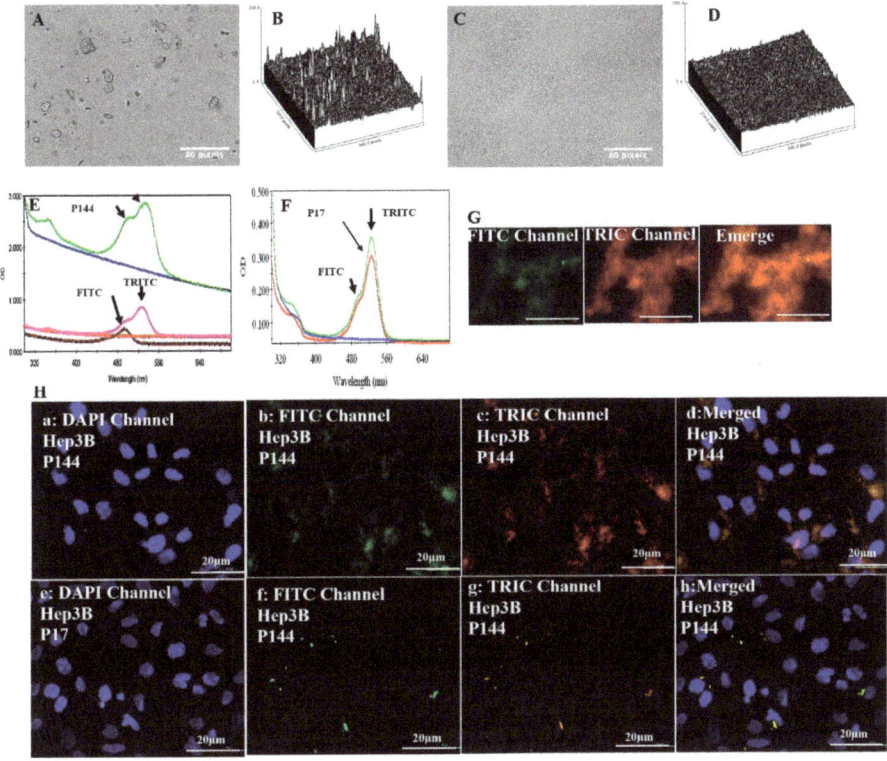

Figure 1. Optical microscopic image of P144 dissolution. (**A**) P144 dissolved by DMSO; (**B**) ImageJ analysis of P144 dissolved by DMSO; (**C**) P144 dissolved by sonication; (**D**) ImageJ analysis of sonicated P144; (**E**) rhodamine-labeled peptide P144; (**F**) rhodamine-labeled peptide P17; (**G**) fluorescence microscopy for images labeled P144. (**H**; **a**–**d**) Cellular uptake of sonicated P144; (**E**–**H**) Cellular uptake of suspended P17.

3.2. Fabrication of Protein–Peptide Mucoadhesive Complex

Both peptides (P17 and 144) were suspended in PBS at pH 7.2 and then P144 was sonicated by ultrasonicator. The processing time was adjusted for 15 min under amplitude five (intensity). The processing time is further divided into three steps each one has taken 5 min. Under magnetic stirrer, the sonicated P144 and suspended P17 were then integrated into BSA moieties in the presence of carbodiimide and n-hydroxy succinimide [33]. The reaction was continued by completing the stirrer for 15 min and then carboxymethyl cellulose was added and the stirring was further continued into addition for 10 min. Free capsules (with no encapsulated peptides) were labeled by fluorescence isothiocyanate (Figure 5 and Supplementary Scheme S1B). Both formulations were then functionalized by adding protamine to observe helix structure [34]. Indeed, protamine can modify the size of particles without any restriction for moieties of the protein–peptide complex. These results showed good turbidity after using protamine due to the presence of arginine (Figure 2A,B) [34]. Peptide protein mucoadhesive nanoparticles exhibit unaggregated and rounded core-shell assembly (Figure 2C–E) and have Z-potential value (−25 mV; Figure 3). This indicates good physical stability of nanosuspensions due to electrostatic repulsion of individual particles. Additionally, folic acid doped carboxymethyl cellulose was added as the last layer to the formulation. This may strengthen the properties of mucoadhesive targeting therapy (Figure 2F,G and Supplementary Scheme S1A). Indeed, this strategy was designed by using two layers from CMC, one is integrated into the middle layer and the second is added as the last layer. Therefore, this mechanism allows facilitating cellular adhesion and penetration, leading to increased stability of peptides in aqueous solution and improved cellular uptake for both peptides (P144 and P17; Supplementary Scheme S2).

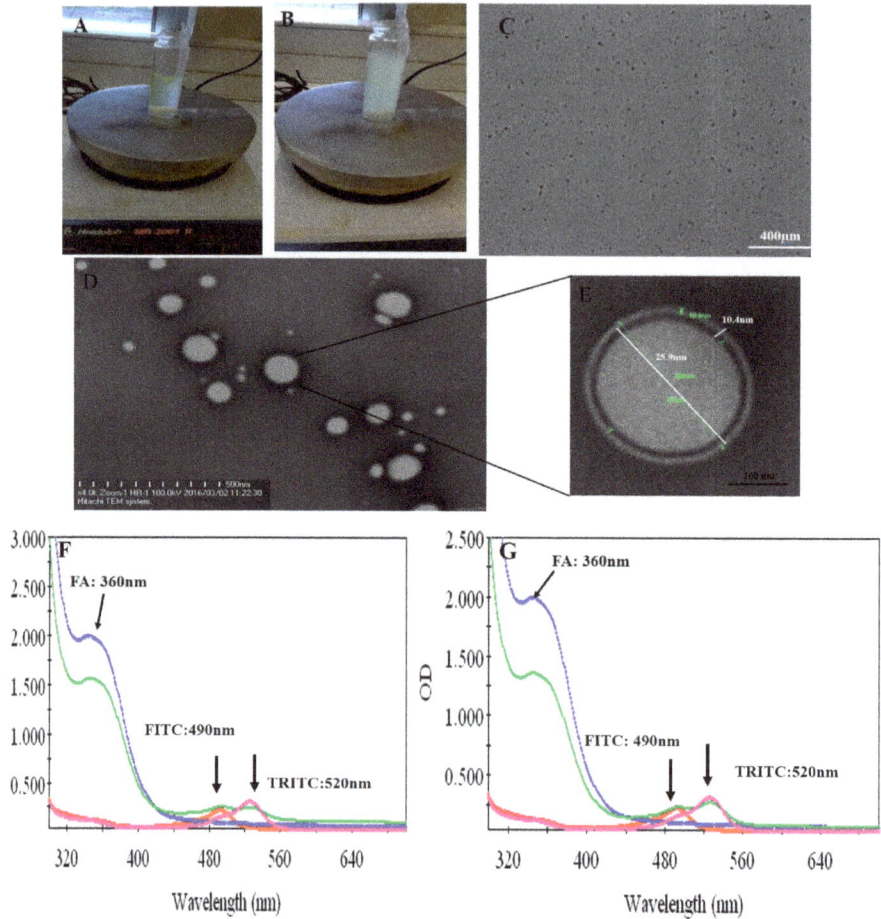

Figure 2. Fabrication of protein–peptide mucoadhesive complex. (**A**) Peptide conjugated protein; (**B**) turbid suspension after adding protamine. (**C**) Optical microscopic image reporting a homogenous distribution of particles. (**D**) Protein–peptide mucoadhesive complex TEM image. (**E**) TEM at high magnification. (**F**) UV–visible absorbance of P17. (**G**) UV–visible absorbance of P144.

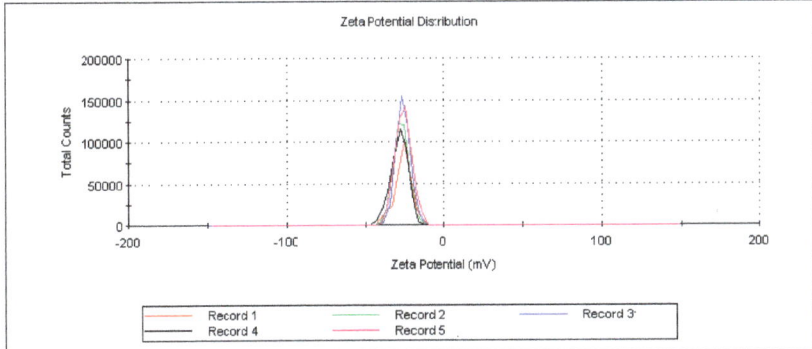

Figure 3. Zeta potential measurement after five successful running data. Each one was run five times with a delay of 5 s after each measurement.

3.3. Biological Experiments: Cellular Uptake

The rhodamine-labeled non-encapsulated peptides were accumulated successfully inside the cytoplasm as shown by fluorescent emission of TRITC channel (red spots). On the other hand, the green color was shown by using the FITC channel, indicating that peptides are able to emit green intensity after their doping with R6G (Figure 1G,H). Similarly, encapsulated peptides that were labeled by rhodamine showed good intensity for both TRITC and FITC channels after their cellular internalization as well (Figure 4A–P). Indeed, the labeled peptides were accumulated around the perinuclear region of both Hep3B and SNU449 cell lines. Such emissions are mostly related to the presence of tryptophan, tyrosine and phenylalanine. While in the presence of rhodamine, the fluorescent signal is strengthened and intensity is increased. It is reported that tryptophan is highly sensitive to hydrogen bonding and non-covalent interactions, displaying a red, green and blue shift [35]. Additionally, its indole group is considered the dominant source of UV absorbance at ~280 nm and emission at ~350 nm [36].

The results indicate that there is a good distribution of adsorbed peptides inside cytoplasm after their encapsulation compared to those used with no encapsulation. Similarly, free capsules were localized inside cytoplasm after their cellular adsorption (Figure 5). On the contrary, the non-encapsulated peptides accumulated in an aggregated state even after their cellular uptake (Figure 1H (merged)). This perhaps explains that the separation of P144 bulk into small particles by using physical sonication is not really enough to keep these particles separately because these particles tend to bind back after their accumulation.

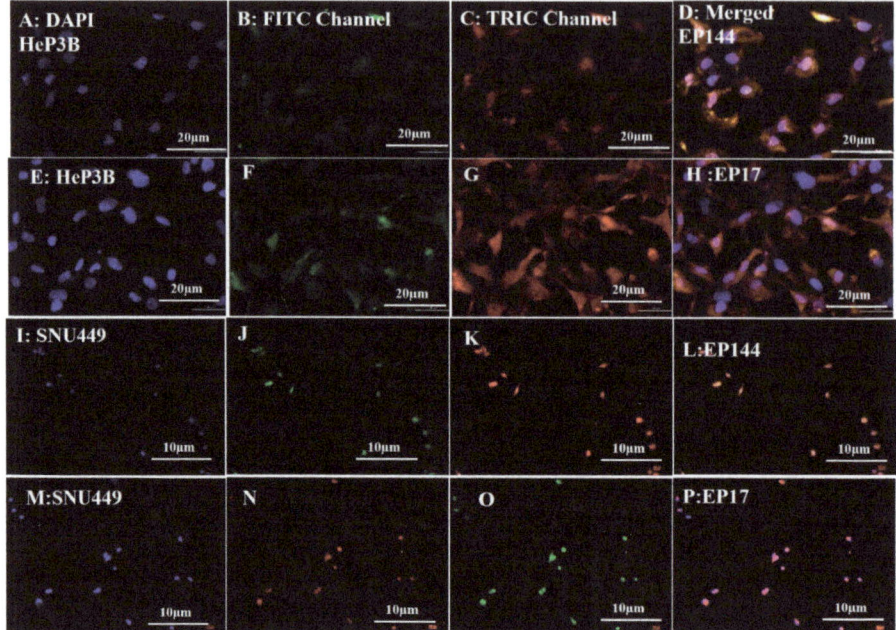

Figure 4. Fluorescence images of cellular uptake (**A–D**) Hep3B adsorbed EP144. (**E–H**) Hep3B adsorbed EP17. (**I–L**) SNU449-adsorbed EP144. (**M–P**) SNU449-adsorbed EP17.

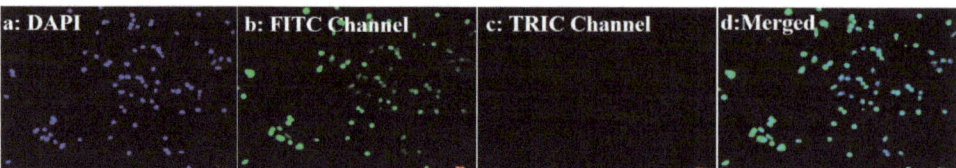

Figure 5. Fluorescence images of cellular uptake. SNU449-adsorbed free capsules.

3.4. Determination of Nuclear Morphology by Using DAPI Staining

DAPI (4', 6-diamidino-2-phenylindole) is a specific fluorophore for a nucleic acid because it is able to bind preferentially to adenine thymine base pair and also to phosphate groups of DNA [37–40]. This mechanism allows researchers to discover the alteration associated with nuclear morphology. In the current study, DAPI staining indicates that there are no changes in nuclear morphology for cells SNU449 after their exposure to 50 µg/mL free capsules (empty vehicles) with no encapsulated peptides for 24 h (Figure 6). However, there are clear alterations for nuclear morphology in both cell lines Hep3B and SNU449 after their exposure to encapsulated P17 and P144 for 24 h. Results showed that there was an increasing number of condensed nuclei, nuclear fragmentation and hypotrophy [41–43]. Additionally, their morphology suffered from phenotype alteration (Figure 7, Part 1 and Part 2).

Pharmaceutics **2020**, *12*, 421

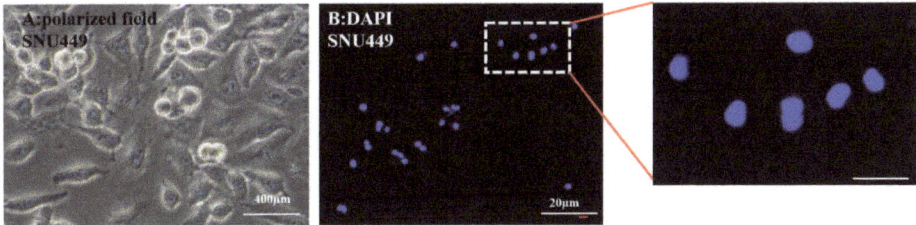

Figure 6. (**A**) Optical microscopy image of SNU449 after their exposure to 50 µg/mL free capsules for 24 h of incubation. (**B**) Fluorescence image of DAPI staining.

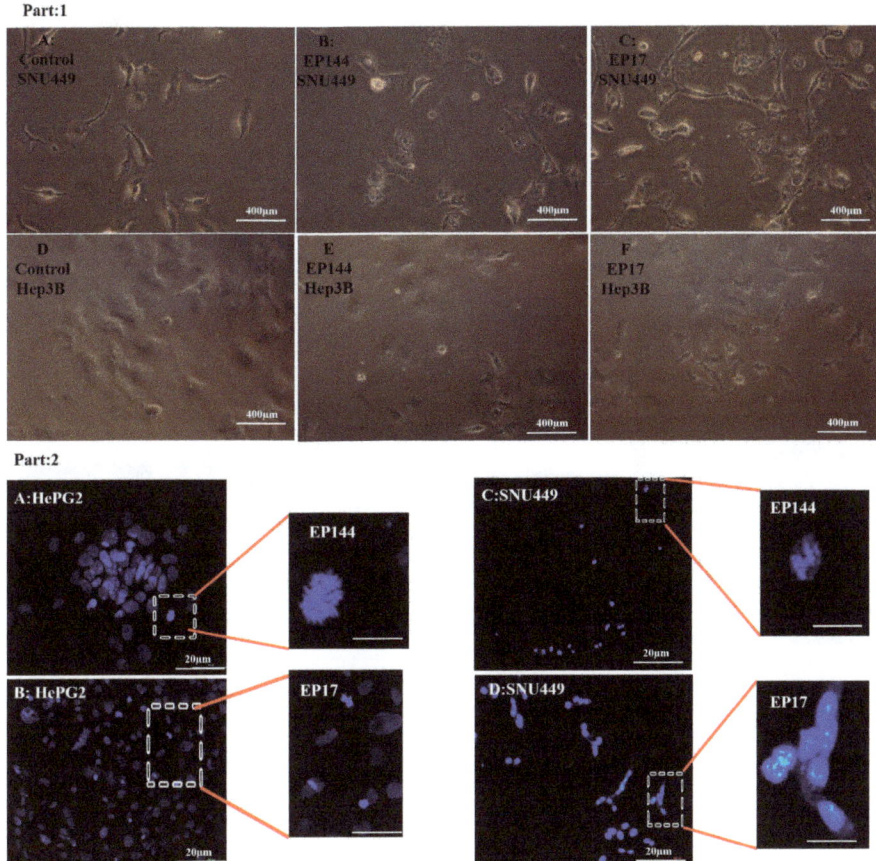

Figure 7. (**Part 1**) SNU449 and Hep3B cell lines suffered from phenotype changes. (**A**) control SNU449. (**B**) SNU449 exposed to 50 µg/mL EP144. (**C**) SNU449 exposed to 50 µg/mL EP17. (**D**) control Hep3B. (**E**) Hep3B exposed to 50 µg/mL EP144. (**F**) Hep3B exposed to 50 µg/mL EP17. (**Part 2**) Fluorescence images of morphology of DAPI staining (**A**) Nuclear degradation at Hep3B. (**B**) Nuclear condensation at Hep3B. (**C**) Nuclear fragmentation at SNU449. (**D**) Nuclear activation at SNU449.

On the contrary, the Hep3B and SNU449 exposed to non-encapsulated peptides exhibited no more changes in their morphology. However, a slightly condensed nucleation was shown (Figure 8, Part 1 and Part 2). Additionally, quantitative analysis of nuclear morphology indicates that Hep3B and SNU449 cells that were exposed to encapsulated peptides (P17 and P144) exhibited significantly nuclear alterations compared to non-encapsulated peptides (Figure 9).

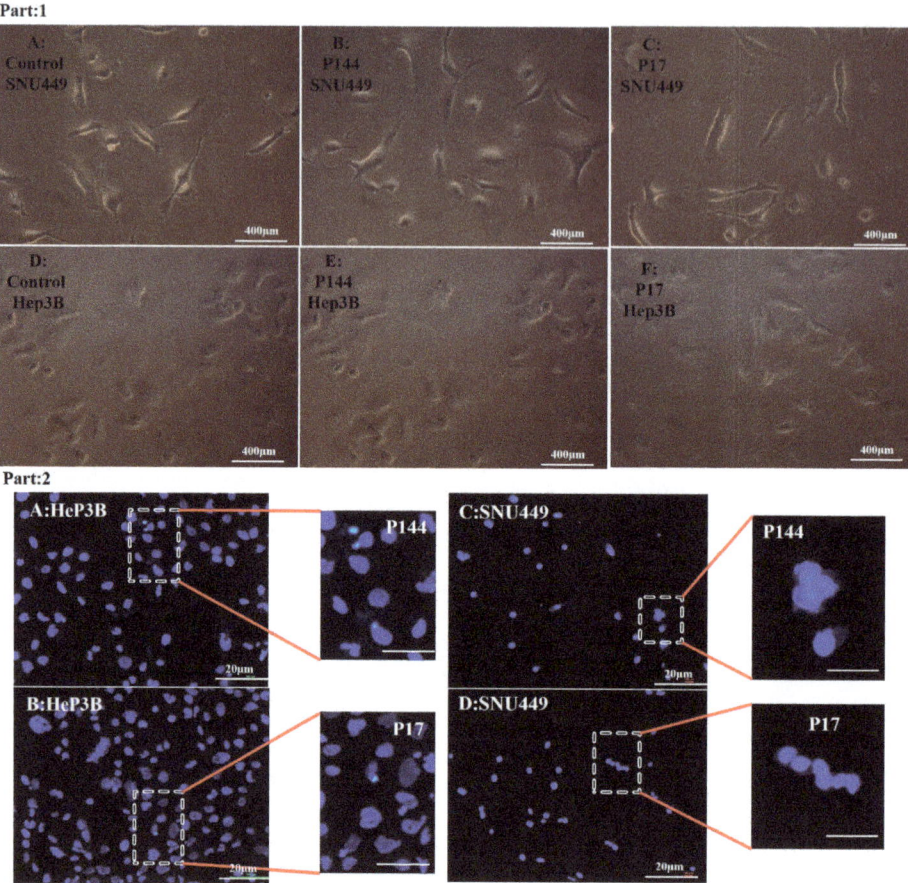

Figure 8. (**Part 1**) Optical microscopy images SNU449 and Hep3B cell lines suffered from phenotype changes. (**A**) control SNU449. (**B**) SNU449 exposed to 50 µg/mL P144. (**C**) SNU449 exposed to 50 µg/mL P17. (**D**) control Hep3B. (**E**) Hep3B exposed to 50 µg/mL P144. (**F**) Hep3B exposed to 50 µg/mL P17. (**Part 2**) Fluorescence images of the morphology of DAPI staining; (**A**) Slightly nuclear condensation at Hep3B. (**B**) Few nuclear condensations. (**C**) Slightly nuclear activation at SNU449. (**D**) No morphological alteration at SNU449.

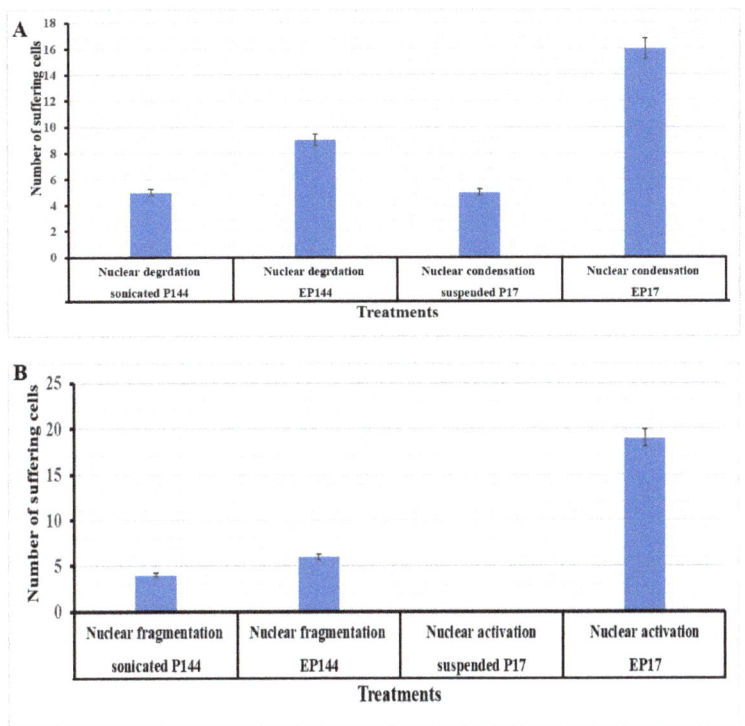

Figure 9. Quantification analysis of nuclear morphology after DAPI staining. (**A**) Hep3B cells exposed to encapsulated and non-encapsulated P17 and P144. (**B**) SNU449 cells exposed to encapsulated and non-encapsulated P17 and P144.

3.5. Antiproliferative Effect of Encapsulated Peptides

Crystal violet cell proliferation assay is a colorimetric method based on the use of crystal violet as a basic dye with avidity to nuclear structures. After binding and solubilization of the crystal violet, optical density measurements of extracted dye provide a measure of the relative number of viable cells. This test has the advantage that it is less time consuming, easier to perform and more objective [29].

Encapsulated peptides (P17 and P144) have an antiproliferative influence on human liver cancer cell lines (SNU449 and Hep3B) as shown by proliferation assay. Both encapsulated peptides (P17 and P144) inhibited the proliferation of human liver cancer cell lines in vitro in a dose-dependent manner. This inhibition was substantial in both cell lines after treatment, with significant differences from 10 µg/mL to 200 µg/mL in treated cells (Figure 10). Similar to our findings, it is reported that P17 and P144 induced antiproliferation effect against human lung cancer cell lines [44] and glioblastoma cell lines [45,46], respectively. On the other hand, Hep3B and SNU449 cell lines exhibited significant proliferation after their exposure to free capsules for 72 h.

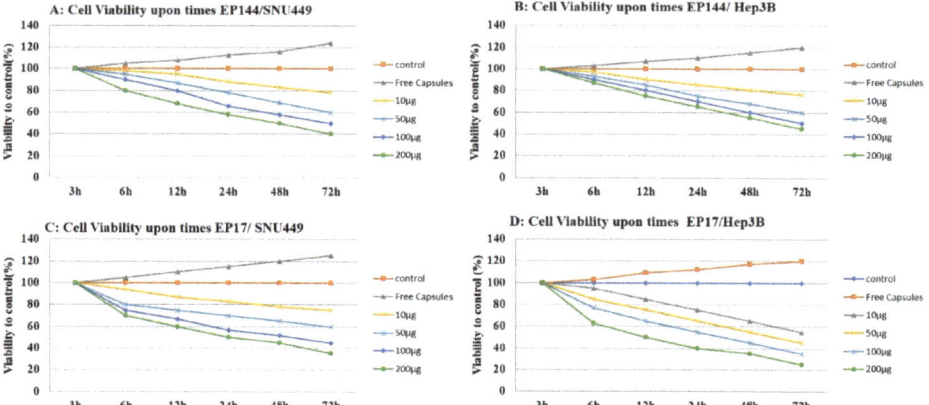

Figure 10. Cell proliferation assay. (**A**) Cell viability of SNU449 in a dose-dependent manner by using different concentrations of encapsulated P144. (**B**) Cell viability of Hep3B in a dose-dependent manner by using different concentrations of encapsulated P144. (**C**) Cell viability of SNU449 in a dose-dependent manner by using different concentrations of encapsulated P17. (**D**) Cell viability of Hep3B in a dose-dependent manner by using different concentrations of encapsulated P17.

3.6. Effects of P144 and P17 on SMAD2 Phosphorylation

SMADs are a group of encoded homologs mammalian protein identified by Small (Sma) and Mothers against dpp (Mad) genes that act as intracellular transcriptional factors [47]. SMAD2 and SMAD3 can be phosphorylated by the TGFβRI after the direct binding of TGFβ ligand to its specific receptors (TGFβRII). This enables them to form heteromeric complexes with SMAD4. This complex is translocated into the nucleus to regulate target genes [48]. Indeed, we next studied the response to TGFβ in terms of SMAD2 phosphorylation in both SNU449 and Hep3B cells. SNU449, but not Hep3B, presented basal SMAD2 phosphorylation. Both cell lines responded to external TGFβ significantly increasing phosphor-SMAD2 levels (Figure 11). Additionally, in the absence of external TGFβ1, SNU449 cells presented lower phosphorylation of SMAD2 after their exposure to P17, but not after their exposure to P144. This phosphorylation was not observed in Hep3B cells after their exposure to P17. However, slight phosphorylation was shown after their exposure to P144. In the presence of external TGFβ1, SNU449 cells increased the pSMAD2 signal after their exposure to P17 and P144. However, Hep3B presented lower phosphorylation of SMAD2 after their exposure to P17, but not after their exposure to P144. Interestingly, in the absence of the external TGFβ1, the encapsulated P17 and P144 caused a reduction of SMAD2 phosphorylation in both SNU449 and Hep3B cells. In presence of the external TGF β1, encapsulated P17 clearly attenuated the level of SMAD2 phosphorylation in Hep3B cells and both encapsulated P144 and P17 attenuated SMAD2 phosphorylation in SNU449 cells. These results indicate that the encapsulation of P17 and P144 clearly shows advantages regarding their biological activity when compared with non-encapsulated peptides, particularly in the mesenchymal, more invasive, SNU449 cell line.

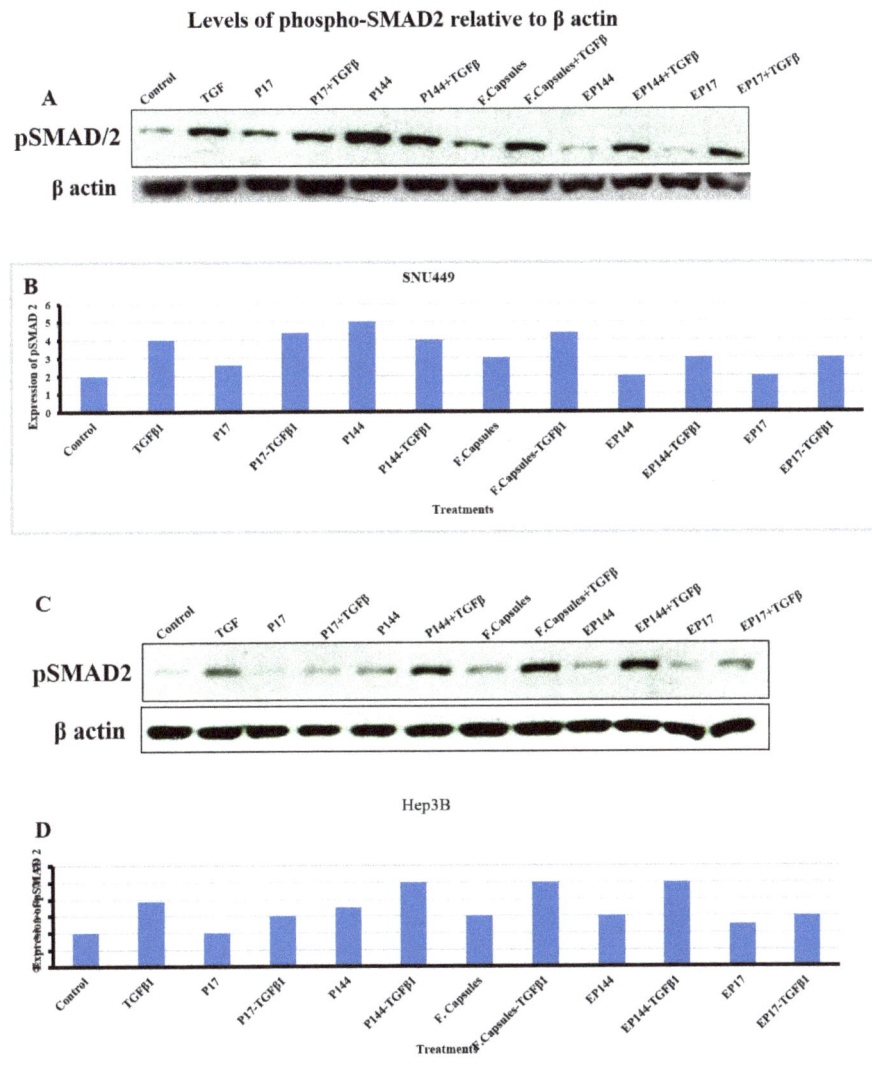

Figure 11. Evaluation of SMAD2 phosphorylation in SNU449 and Hep3B cells. (**A,C**) Western blot band of pSMAD2; beta-actin was analyzed as loading control. (**B,D**) Densitometric analysis of pSMAD2 levels after their exposure to several treatments for 6 h.

4. Discussion

TGFβ1 inhibitory peptides have attracted much interest recently because of their ability to block the TGFβ1 signaling pathway [49], due to their possible binding to the extracellular region where the TGFβ1 ligand connects with its cellular receptors [30]. It is reported previously that the bulk of P144 can be separated into small particles by using sonication [30]. However, these small particles tend to be aggregated. This action may attribute their loss of the physicochemical interaction after sonication. Such action leads to the distribution of the electrostatic balance among these particles. For this reason, the small particles tend to be aggregated back after their separation. In the current work, we analyzed the possible separation of these particles by the next interaction with BSA. Hence, these particles are integrated into the moieties of BSA. This coupled interaction drives keeping the small particles of peptides under electrostatic balance and preventing their aggregation. The demonstration of rhodamine-labeled peptides exhibited a specific peak at 550 nm which is attributed to the main peak of pure rhodamine [32]. Increasingly, the second peak was shown at 490 nm, which is similar to the main peaks of fluorescent isocyanate [50]. Perhaps, the central carbon atom of the chromophore is influenced by the ionic stress of the complex leading to a shift of both absorption and fluorescence emission related to the presence of tryptophan [35]. Rhodamine-labeled peptides advanced our knowledge concerning the physicochemical properties of these two peptides. For instance, their aggregation was localized even after their cellular uptake around the cytoplasmic region. This evidence was first detected by using fluorescence microscopy after their precipitation upon the surface of the slide (Figure 1G). In the same way, small particles of both peptides were compacted after their internalization with no equal distribution in the perinuclear region. To evaluate their aggregation, ImageJ analysis was used and it refers to the presence of an aggregation state in non-encapsulated peptides compared to encapsulated peptides (Supplementary Materials, Figure S1).

The protein–peptide assembly was further functionalized by protamine sulfate. This provides a novel strategy in terms of α helix titration resulting in turbidity [34]. Arginine rich protamine is responsible for this turbidity and it perhaps causes modification to the diameter of nanoparticles [51]. Furthermore, there is no published report observing immune-stimulatory side effects related to the use of protamine [51,52]. To increase their adhesion and cellular adsorption, this complex was further functionalized by folic acid conjugated carboxymethyl cellulose.

Apart from cellular adsorption, the DAPI staining noticeably revealed nuclear morphological changes in both SNU449 and Hep3B human liver cancer cell lines in terms of nuclear fragmentation, nuclear hypotrophy, nuclear condensation and cell structure loss. Accordingly, the present results proved significantly the potential efficient therapy of both encapsulated peptides against the analyzed cell lines. Similar to our results, P144 and P17 treatment resulted in significant inhibition at lung cancer cell lines [44] and the growth of glioblastoma cell lines [46] respectively. When analyzing the effects of encapsulated versus non-encapsulated peptides at the cellular level, we observed that the efficiency of the encapsulated peptides was remarkably higher in the SNU449 cells. We and other authors had previously demonstrated that the SNU449 cells show autocrine stimulation of the TGFβ pathway and respond to TGF-β increasing Smad2/3 phosphorylation [53]. These cells are resistant to the suppressor effects of TGFβ [54] and respond to it undergoing EMT. Here, we show that encapsulated peptides (P17 and P144) induced significant inhibition of basal pSMAD2 in SNU449 cells when compared to non-encapsulated peptides. Additionally, pSMAD2 phosphorylation is considerably attenuated after TGFβ treatment. In summary, the transforming growth factor β (TGF-β) signaling pathway consists of extracellular ligands (including the TGF-β-like group and BMP-like group). The TGF-β-like group generally phosphorylates SMAD2 and SMAD3, whereas the BMP-like group generally induces phosphorylation of SMAD1, SMAD5 and SAMD8 [55]. The activated R-SMADs form hetero-oligomeric complexes with Co-SMAD (SMAD4), which are translocated to the nucleus where they regulate the expression of target genes. In general, both pathways are translocated into the nucleus to translate the signal [56]. In this recent study, the phosphorylation of SMAD2 was studied using Western blot analysis. Additionally, nuclear alteration was distinguished.

5. Conclusions

In conclusion, the encapsulation of TGFβ inhibitory peptides (P17 and P144) has shown potential therapeutic inhibition to basal phospho-SMAD as a result of TGF-β pathway regulation. It has proved clearly their ability to inhibit the autocrine TGFβ pathway and basal nuclear SMAD. However, SNU449 is one of the cell lines that is more responsive to those encapsulated by P17 and P144 is a mesenchymal, invasive HCC cell line that produces TGFβ autocrinally and is unresponsive to its suppressor effects. Additionally, rhodamine-labeled peptides enable researchers to follow nearly the localization of peptides inside cytoplasm after their cellular uptake. In the current studies and our previous studies indicated that encapsulation of TGFβ signaling pathway inhibitors may facilitate their delivery and overcome their cytotoxicity. Additionally, folic acid functionalized drug delivery systems enable them to reach and accumulate inside cancer cells [57–62].

Supplementary Materials: The following are available online at http://www.mdpi.com/1999-4923/12/5/421/s1, Figure S1: Fluorescence microscopy images for labelled P144, Scheme S1: (A): Folic Acid conjugated carboxymethyl cellulose. (B) Labelling carboxymethyl cellulose with FITC, Scheme S2: Fabrication of protein mucoadhesive targeted therapy.

Author Contributions: Formal analysis, M.E.K.; funding acquisition, S.L., I.F.; investigation and analysis, N.A.N.H.; methodology, N.A.N.H.; supervision, I.F., S.L. and M.E.K.; writing—original draft, N.A.N.H., revised by I.F. and S.L. All authors have read and agreed to the published version of the manuscript.

Funding: This work was supported by REA Research Grant n. PITN-GA-2012-316549 (IT LIVER) from the People Programme (Marie Curie Actions) of the European Union's Seventh Framework Programme (FP7/2007–2013). S.L. is supported by Progetto FISR-CNR "Tecnopolo di Nanotecnologia e Fotonica per la Medicina di Precisione"- CUP B83B17000010001.

Acknowledgments: This work was supported by Institute of Nanoscience and Nanotechnology, Kafrelsheikh University, Egypt.

Conflicts of Interest: The authors declare no conflict of interest

References

1. David, C.J.; Massague, J. Contextual determinants of TGF-ß action in development, immunity and cancer. *Nat. Rev. Mol. Cell Biol.* **2018**, *19*, 419–435. [CrossRef] [PubMed]
2. Miyazawa, K.; Miyazono, K. Regulation of TGF- ß family signaling by inhibitory SMADs. *Cold Spring Harb. Perspect. Biol.* **2017**, *9*, a022095.
3. Hanafy, N.A.; El Kemary, M. TGFβ1 as a Good and Bad Biological Molecule: Structure and Function. *Biomed. J. Sci. Tech. Res. BJSTR* **2019**. [CrossRef]
4. Landén, N.X.; Li, D.; Ståhle, M. Transition from inflammation to proliferation: A critical step during wound healing. *Cell. Mol. Life Sci.* **2016**, *73*, 3861–3885.
5. Zhang, Y.; Alexander, P.B.; Wang, X.F. TGF- ß family signaling in the control of cell proliferation and survival. *Cold Spring Harb. Perspect. Biol.* **2017**, *9*, a022145. [CrossRef]
6. ten Dijke, P.; Arthur, H.M. Extracellular control of TGF-ß beta signalling in vascular development and disease. *Nat. Rev. Mol. Cell Biol.* **2007**, *8*, 857–869. [CrossRef]
7. Heldin, C.H.; Moustakas, A. Signaling receptors for TGF-ß family members. *Cold Spring Harb. Perspect. Biol.* **2016**, *8*, a022053. [CrossRef]
8. Zarranz-Ventura, J.; Fernández-Robredo, P.; Recalde, S.; Salinas-Alamán, A.; Borrás-Cuesta, F.; Dotor, J.; García-Layana, A. Transforming growth factor-beta inhibition reduces progression of early choroidal neovascularization lesions in rats: P17 and P144 peptides. *PLoS ONE* **2013**, *31*, e65434. [CrossRef]
9. Murillo-Cuesta, S.; Rodríguez-de la Rosa, L.; Contreras, J.; Celaya, A.M.; Camarero, G.; Rivera, T.; Varela-Nieto, I. Transforming growth factor β1 inhibition protects from noise-induced hearing loss. *Front. Aging Neurosci.* **2015**, *7*, 32.
10. Ezquerro, I.J.; Lasarte, J.J.; Dotor, J. A synthetic peptide from transforming growth factor β type III receptor inhibits liver fibrogenesis in rats with carbon tetrachloride liver injury. *Cytokine* **2003**, *22*, 12–20. [CrossRef]
11. Dotor, J.; Lopez-Vazquez, A.B.; Lasarte, J.J.; Sarobe, P.; Garcia-Granero, M.; Riezu-Boj, J.I.; Martinez, A.; Feijoo, E.; Lopez-Sagaseta, J.; Hermida, J.; et al. Identification of peptide inhibitors of transforming growth factor beta 1 using a phage displayed peptide library. *Cytokine* **2007**, *39*, 106–115. [CrossRef] [PubMed]
12. Gil-Guerrero, L.; Dotor, J.; Huibregtse, I.J.; Casares, N.; Lopez-Vazquez, A.B.; Rudilla, F.; Riezu-Boj, J.I.; Lopez-Sagaseta, J.; Hermida, J.; Van Deventer, S.; et al. In vitro and in vivo down-regulation of regulatory T-cell activity with a peptide inhibitor of TGF-beta1. *J. Immunol.* **2008**, *181*, 126–135.
13. Santiago, B.; Gutierrez-Canas, I.; Dotor, J.; Palao, G.; Lasarte, J.J.; Ruiz, J.; Prieto, J.; Borras-Cuesta, F.; Pablos, J.L. Topical application of a peptide inhibitor of transforming growth factor-beta1 ameliorates bleomycin-induced skin fibrosis. *J. Investig. Dermatol.* **2005**, *125*, 450–455. [CrossRef] [PubMed]

14. Kratz, F.; Müller-Driver, R.; Hofmann, I.; Drevs, J.; Unger, C. A novel macromolecular prodrug concept exploiting endogenous serum albumin as a drug carrier for cancer chemotherapy. *J. Med. Chem.* **2000**, *43*, 1253–1256. [CrossRef]
15. Llopiz, D.; Dotor, J.; Zabaleta, A.; Lasarte, J.J.; Prieto, J.; Borras-Cuesta, F.; Sarobe, P. Combined immunization with adjuvant molecules poly(I:C) and anti-CD40 plus a tumour antigen has potent prophylactic and therapeutic antitumor effects. *Cancer Immunol. Immunother.* **2008**, *57*, 19–29. [CrossRef] [PubMed]
16. Recalde, S.; Zarranz-Ventura, J.; Fernández-Robredo, P.; García-Gómez, P.J.; Salinas-Alamán, A.; Borrás-Cuesta, F.; Dotor, J.; García-Layana, A. Transforming growth factor-β inhibition decreases diode laser-induced choroidal neovascularization development in rats: P17 and P144 peptides. *Investig. Ophthalmol. Vis. Sci.* **2011**, *52*, 7090–7097. [CrossRef] [PubMed]
17. Qiu, S.S.; Dotor, J.; Hontanilla, B. Effect of P144® (Anti-TGF-β) in an "In Vivo" Human Hypertrophic Scar Model in Nude Mice. *PLoS ONE* **2015**, *10*, e0144489. [CrossRef]
18. Da Violante, G.; Zerrouk, N.; Richard, I.; Provot, G.; Chaumeil, J.C.; Arnaud, P. Evaluation of the cytotoxicity effect of dimethyl sulfoxide (DMSO) on Caco2/TC7 colon tumor cell cultures. *Biol. Pharm. Bull.* **2002**, *25*, 1600–1603. [CrossRef]
19. Hanafy, N.A.N. Encapsulation of cancer signalling pathway inhibitors as a protective way for healthy cells. Commentary. *Med. Res. Innov.* **2018**. [CrossRef]
20. Soukupova, J.; Malfettone, A.; Hyrošš ová, P.; Hernández-Alvarez, M.I.; Peñuelas-Haro, I.; Bertran, E.; Junza, A.; Capellades, J.; Giannelli, G.; Yanes, O.; et al. Role of the Transforming Growth Factor-β in regulating hepatocellular carcinoma oxidative metabolism. *Sci. Rep.* **2017**, *7*, 12486. [CrossRef]
21. American Type Culture Collection. Available online: www.lgcstandards-atcc.org (accessed on 5 November 2018).
22. Zhou, Q.Y.; Tu, C.Y.; Shao, C.X.; Wang, W.K.; Zhu, J.D.; Cai, Y.; Mao, J.Y.; Chen, W. GC7 blocks epithelial-mesenchymal transition and reverses hypoxia-induced chemotherapy resistance in hepatocellular carcinoma cells. *Am. J. Transl. Res.* **2017**, *9*, 2608–2617. [PubMed]
23. Hanafy, N.A.N.; El-Kemary, M.; Leporatti, S. Reduction diameter of $CaCO_3$ crystals by using poly acrylic acid might improve cellular uptake of encapsulated curcumin in breast cancer. *J. Nanomed. Res.* **2018**, *7*, 235–239.
24. Hanafy, N.A.N.; Ferraro, M.M.; Gaballo, A.; Dini, L.; Tasco, V.; Nobile, C.; De Giorgi, M.L.; Carallo, S.; Rinaldi, R.; Leporatti, S. Fabrication and Characterization of ALK1fc-Loaded Fluoro-Magnetic Nanoparticles Rods for Inhibiting TGF β1 in HCC. *RSC Adv.* **2016**, *6*, 48834–48842. [CrossRef]
25. Hanafy, N.A.N.; El-Kemary, M.; Leporatti, S. Mucoadhesive curcumin crosslinked carboxy methyl cellulose might increase inhibitory efficiency for liver cancer treatment. *Mater. Sci. Eng. C* **2020**, in press.
26. Safer, A.M.; Sen, A.; Hanafy, N.A.; Mousa, S.A. Quantification of the healing effect in hepatic fibrosis induced by Chitosan Nano-encapsulated Green Tea in Rat Model Studied—At Ultrastructural level. *J. Nanosci. Nanotechnol.* **2015**, *15*, 1–7.
27. Hanafy, N.A.; Nobile, C.; De Giorgi, M.L.; Ran, B.; Cao, Y.; Giannelli, G.; Leporatti, S. LY2157299-Loaded Carriers Inhibiting Wound Healing in Hepatocellular Carcinoma. *J. Biotech.* **2014**, *185S*, S18–S36. [CrossRef]
28. Hanafy, N.A.N.; De Giorgi, M.L.; Nobile, C.; Giannelli, G.; Quarta, A.; Leporatti, S. P0253: Inhibition of glycolysis by using nano lipid bromopyruvic chitosan carrier is a promising tool to prevent HCC invasiveness. *J. Hepatol.* **2015**, *62*, S401. [CrossRef]
29. Chiba, K.; Kawakami, K.; Tohyama, K. Simultaneous evaluation of cell viability by neutral red, MTT and crystal violet staining assays of the same cells. *Toxicol. Vitro* **1998**, *12*, 251–258. [CrossRef]
30. Hanafy, N.A.N.; Quarta, A.; Di Corato, R.; Dini, L.; Nobile, C.; De Giorgi, M.L.; Tasco, V.; Carallo, S.; Cascione, M.; Rinaldi, R.; et al. Encapsulation of SHT-DNA, SIRNA and polypeptide -17 inside Hybrid polymeric nano-protein folic acid (HPNP-FA) carriers as targeted TGF beta inhibitor for Hepatocellular carcinoma. *J. Hepatol.* **2016**, *64*, S425–S630. [CrossRef]
31. Jang, C.W.; Chen, C.H.; Chen, C.C.; Chen, J.; Su, Y.H.; Chen, R.H. TGF-β induces apoptosis through Smad-mediated expression of DAP-kinase. *Nat. Cell Biology* **2002**, *4*, 51–58. [CrossRef]
32. Beija, M.; Afonso, C.A.M.; Martinho, J.M.G. Synthesis and applications of Rhodamine derivatives as fluorescent probes. *Chem. Soc. Rev.* **2009**, *38*, 2410–2433. [CrossRef] [PubMed]
33. Parodi, A.; Miao, J.; Soond, S.M.; Rudzińska, M.R.; Zamyatnin, A.A. Albumin Nanovectors in Cancer Therapy and Imaging. *Biomolecules* **2019**, *9*, 218. [CrossRef] [PubMed]

34. Scheicher, B.; Lorenzer, C.; Gegenbauer, K.; Partlic, J.; Andreae, F.; Kirsch, A.H.; Rosenkranz, A.R.; Werzer, O.; Zimmer, A. Manufacturing of a Secretoneurin Drug Delivery System with Self-Assembled Protamine Nanoparticles by Titration. *PLoS ONE* **2016**, *11*, e0164149. [CrossRef] [PubMed]
35. Piston, D.W.; Kremers, G.J. Fluorescent protein FRET: The good, the bad and the ugly. *Trends Biochem. Sci.* **2007**, *32*, 407–414. [CrossRef] [PubMed]
36. Teale, F.W.J.; Weber, G. Ultraviolet fluorescence of the aromatic amino acids. *Biochem. J.* **1957**, *65*, 476–482. [CrossRef]
37. Junghans, M.; Kreuter, J.; Zimmer, A. Antisense delivery using protamine-oligonucleotide particles. *Nucleic Acids Res.* **2000**, *28*, e45. [CrossRef]
38. Kubista, M.; Aakerman, B.; Norden, B. Characterization of interaction between DNA and 4′,6-diamidino-2-phenylindole by optical spectroscopy. *Biochemistry* **1987**, *26*, 4545–4553. [CrossRef]
39. Barcellona, M.L.; Favilla, R.; Von Berger, J.; Avitabile, M.; Ragusa, N.; Masotti, L. DNA-4′-6-diamidine-2-phenylindole interactions: A comparative study employing fluorescence and ultraviolet spectroscopy. *Arch. Biochem. Biophys.* **1986**, *250*, 48–53. [CrossRef]
40. Kntayya, S.B.; Ibrahim, D.M.; Ain, M.N.; Iori, R.; Ioannides, C.; Abdull Razis, A.F. Induction of Apoptosis and Cytotoxicity by Isothiocyanate Sulforaphene in Human Hepatocarcinoma HepG2 Cells. *Nutrients* **2018**, *10*, 718. [CrossRef]
41. Estandarte, A.K.; Botchway, S.; Lynch, C.; Yusuf, M.; Robinson, I. The use of DAPI fluorescence lifetime imaging for investigating chromatin condensation in human chromosomes. *Sci. Rep.* **2016**, *16*, 31417. [CrossRef]
42. Gallo-Oller, G.; Vollmann-Zwerenz, A.; Melendez, B.; Rey, J.; Hau, P.; Dotor, J.; Castresana, J. P144, a Transforming Growth Factor beta inhibitor peptide, generates antitumoral effects and modifies SMAD7 and SKI levels in human glioblastoma cell lines. *Cancer Lett.* **2016**, *381*, 67–75. [CrossRef] [PubMed]
43. Llopiz, D.; Dotor, J.; Casares, N.; Bezunartea, J.; Díaz-Valdés, N.; Ruiz, M.; Aranda, F.; Berraondo, P.; Prieto, J.; Lasarte, J.J.; et al. Peptide inhibitors of transforming growth factor-beta enhance the efficacy of antitumor immunotherapy. *Int. J. Cancer* **2009**, *125*, 2614–2623. [CrossRef] [PubMed]
44. Zhang, J.; Pan, Y.; Liao, D.; Tang, J.; Yao, D. Peptide 17, an inhibitor of YAP/TEAD4 pathway, mitigates lung cancer malignancy. *Trop. J. Pharm. Res.* **2018**, *17*, 1256. [CrossRef]
45. Upadhyay, A.; Moss-Taylor, L.; Kim, M.J.; Ghosh, A.C.; O'Connor, M.B. TGF-β family signaling in drosophila. *Cold Spring Harb. Perspect. Biol.* **2017**, *9*, a022152. [CrossRef]
46. Savage-Dunn, C.; Padgett, R.W. The TGFβ family in caenorhabditis elegans. *Cold Spring Harb. Perspect. Biol.* **2017**, *9*, a022178. [CrossRef]
47. Hao, Y.; Baker, D.; ten Dijke, P. TGFβ-Mediated Epithelial-Mesenchymal Transition and Cancer Metastasis. *Int. J. Mol. Sci.* **2019**, *20*, 2767. [CrossRef]
48. Hanafy, N.A.N.; Quarta, A.; Di Corato, R.; Dini, L.; Nobile, C.; Tasco, V.; Carallo, S.; Cascione, M.; Malfettone, A.; Soukupova, J.; et al. Hybrid polymeric-protein nano-carriers (HPPNC) for targeted delivery of TGFβ inhibitors to hepatocellular carcinoma cells. *J. Mater. Sci. Mater. Med.* **2017**, *28*, 120. [CrossRef]
49. Hanafy, N.A.; De Giorgi, M.L.; Nobile, C.; Rinaldi, R.; Leporatti, S. Control of Colloidal CaCO$_3$ suspension by using biodegradable polymers during fabrication. *Beni-Suef Univ. J. Basic Appl. Sci.* **2015**, *4*, 60–70.
50. Chaganti, L.K.; Venkatakrishnan, N.; Bose, K. An efficient method for FITC labelling of proteins using tandem affinity purification. *Biosci. Rep.* **2018**, *38*. [CrossRef]
51. Takikawa, M.; Nakamura, S.; Ishihara, M.; Takabayashi, Y.; Fujita, M.; Hattori, H. Improved angiogenesis and healing in crush syndrome by fibroblast growth factor-2 containing low-molecular-weight heparin (Fragmin)/protamine nanoparticles. *J. Surg. Res.* **2015**, *196*, 247–257. [CrossRef]
52. Mayer, G.; Vogel, V.; Weyermann, J.; Lochmann, D.; van den Broek, J.A.; Tziatzios, C. Oligonucleotideprotamine- albumin nanoparticles: Protamine sulfate causes drastic size reduction. *J. Control. Release* **2005**, *106*, 181–187. [CrossRef] [PubMed]
53. Malfettone, A.; Soukupova, J.; Bertran, E.; Crosas-Molist, E.; Lastra, R.; Fernando, J.; Koudelkova, P.; Rani, B.; Fabra, Á.; Serrano, T.; et al. Transforming growth factor-β-induced plasticity causes a migratory stemness phenotype in hepatocellular carcinoma. *Cancer Lett.* **2017**, *392*, 39–50. [CrossRef] [PubMed]

54. Bertran, E.; Crosas-Molist, E.; Sancho, P.; Caja, L.; Lopez-Luque, J.; Navarro, E.; Egea, G.; Lastra, R.; Serrano, T.; Ramos, E.; et al. Overactivation of the TGF-β pathway confers a mesenchymal-like phenotype and CXCR4-dependent migratory properties to liver tumor cells. *Hepatology* **2013**, *58*, 2032–2044. [CrossRef] [PubMed]
55. Hata, A.; Chen, Y.G. TGF-β signaling from receptors to smads. *Cold Spring Harb. Perspect. Biol.* **2016**, *8*, a022061. [CrossRef] [PubMed]
56. Zheng, S.; Long, J.; Liu, Z.; Tao, W.; Wang, D. Identification and Evolution of TGF-β Signaling Pathway Members in Twenty-Four Animal Species and Expression in Tilapia. *Int. J. Mol. Sci.* **2018**, *19*, 1154. [CrossRef] [PubMed]
57. Hanafy, N.A.; Dini, L.; Citti, C.; Cannazza, G.; Leporatti, S. Inhibition of Glycolysis by Using a Micro/Nano-Lipid Bromopyruvic Chitosan Carrier as a Promising Tool to Improve Treatment of Hepatocellular Carcinoma. *Nanomaterials* **2018**, *8*, 34. [CrossRef]
58. Hanafy, N.A.; De Giorgi, M.L.; Nobile, C.; Cascione, M.; Rinaldi, R.; Leporatti, S. CaCO3 rods as chitosan polygalacturonic acid carriers for brompyruvic acid delivery. *Sci. Adv. Mater.* **2016**, *8*, 514–523. [CrossRef]
59. Hanafy, N.A.N. The growth of hepatocellular carcinoma can be inhibited by encapsulation of TGF ß1 antagonists. *SL Pharmacol. Toxicol.* **2018**, *1*, 112.
60. Hanafy, N.A.N.; El-Kemary, M.; Leporatti, S. Understanding TGF β1 signalling pathway is well strategy to use its encapsulated antagonist as nano therapeutic molecules. *Transl. Sci.* **2018**, *2018*.
61. Hanafy, N.A.N. Glycolysis is a promising target for encapsulation nano-therapeutic molecules against cancer cells. Commentary. *Integr. Cancer Sci. Therap.* **2017**, *2017*.
62. Hanafy, N.A.N. Development and Production of Multifunctional Bio-Nano-Engineered Drug Delivery Systems Loaded by TGF Inhibitors for Delivering into Hepatocellular Carcinoma Cells. Ph.D. Thesis, Salento University Italy, Lecce, Italy, 2017.

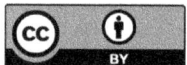

© 2020 by the authors. Licensee MDPI, Basel, Switzerland. This article is an open access article distributed under the terms and conditions of the Creative Commons Attribution (CC BY) license (http://creativecommons.org/licenses/by/4.0/).

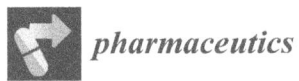

Article

Crosslinked Hyaluronan Electrospun Nanofibers for Ferulic Acid Ocular Delivery

Maria Aurora Grimaudo *, Angel Concheiro and Carmen Alvarez-Lorenzo *

Departamento de Farmacología, Farmacia y Tecnología Farmacéutica, I+D Farma (GI-1645), Facultad de Farmacia and Health Research Institute of Santiago de Compostela (IDIS), Universidade de Santiago de Compostela, 15782-Santiago de Compostela, Spain; angel.concheiro@usc.es

* Correspondence: Maria.Aurora.Grimaudo@sergas.es (M.A.G.); carmen.alvarez.lorenzo@usc.es (C.A.-L.); Tel.: +34-881815239 (M.A.G.)

Received: 20 January 2020; Accepted: 11 March 2020; Published: 17 March 2020

Abstract: Electrospun nanofibers are gaining interest as ocular drug delivery platforms that may adapt to the eye surface and provide sustained release. The aim of this work was to design an innovative ophthalmic insert composed of hyaluronan (HA) nanofibers for the dual delivery of an antioxidant (ferulic acid, FA) and an antimicrobial peptide (ε-polylysine, ε-PL). Polyvinylpyrrolidone (PVP) was added to facilitate the electrospinning process. Fibers with diameters of approx. 100 nm were obtained with PVP 5%-HA 0.8% w/v and PVP 10%-HA 0.5% w/v mixtures in ethanol:water 4:6 v/v. An increase in PVP concentration to 20% w/v in both presence and absence of HA rendered fibers of approx. 1 μm. PVP 5%-HA 0.8% w/v fibers were loaded with 83.3 ± 14.0 μg FA per mg. After nanofibers crosslinking with ε-PL, blank and FA-loaded inserts showed a mean thickness of 270 ± 21 μm and 273 ± 41 μm, respectively. Blank and FA-loaded inserts completely released ε-PL within 30 min under sink conditions, whereas FA-loaded inserts released the antioxidant within 20 min. Both blank and FA-loaded inserts were challenged against *Pseudomonas aeruginosa* and *Staphylococcus aureus*, demonstrating their efficacy against relevant microbial species.

Keywords: ocular inserts; electrospinning; hyaluronan; ferulic acid; ε-polylysine; nanofibers

1. Introduction

Electrospinning is becoming a popular technique due to the mild processing conditions and the versatility of substances that can be processed [1]. It may allow manufacturing polymeric fibers with diameter in the nanoscale in a controllable and cost-effective manner with minimum waste of materials [2–4]. Electrospun fibers characteristics (diameter, surface properties) can be controlled by tuning process variables (applied voltage, solution flow rate, distance between charged capillary and collector) and polymer variety (MW) and solution properties (composition, viscosity, surface tension, solvent volatility, conductivity, and surface charge density) [1,5]. Electrospun fiber shaped nanostructures have high surface area-to-volume ratio and tunable porosity [2], which may resemble the extracellular matrix. Therefore, this technique has been widely explored for tissue engineering and regenerative medicine applications [6–8].

Although less investigated, electrospun nanofibers of natural and synthetic polymers may also find applications as drug delivery platforms, particularly in those cases that thin devices with high specific surface area are required to facilitate the delivery of poorly soluble drugs [9,10]. Drug amorphization in electrospun materials have been proposed to achieve flash or immediate release [11]. Combinations of hydrophilic and hydrophobic polymers and coatings with functional materials have been also tested for endowing the nanofibers with controlled release capabilities [12].

In the ocular field, electrospun nanofibers are gaining interest as soft materials that can easily adapt to cornea and sclera surfaces and remain on the eye surface for a moderate period of time acting as sustained release platforms [13–15]. Thus, compared to liquid and semisolid formulations, electrospun inserts may overcome better the precorneal barriers that oppose to ocular bioavailability after topical application [16]. Increased precorneal residence time and higher and prolonged levels of drugs in the aqueous humor have been observed by using nanofibers [17–19]. Moreover, nanofibers may create a stable transmembrane drug gradient that facilitates the diffusion through the ocular structures of both hydrophilic and lipophilic drugs [14,20–25].

Hyaluronic acid (HA, Figure 1) is a widely used biopolymer in drug delivery and regenerative field due to its biocompatibility, biodegradability and wound healing properties [26]. This negatively charged glycosaminoglycan, composed of alternating units of D-glucuronic acid and N-acetyl-D-glucosamine, can be hardly electrospun from aqueous solutions due to the high surface tension and chain stiffness that results from the long electrostatic interactions and intramolecular hydrogen bonds, increasing the viscosity. For these reasons, HA has been electrospun in association with other polymers [27–29].

Polyvinylpyrrolidone (PVP, Figure 1), another Generally Recognized as Safe (GRAS) excipient, also shows excellent water solubility, biological compatibility, film forming and bioadhesion features [30]. Conversely to HA, PVP nanofibers can be easily electrospun from aqueous solutions [31], although the fibers exhibit rapid disintegration in physiological fluids [32].

Green or natural crosslinking agents have been proposed to prepare HA networks [33]. ε-polylysine (ε-PL, Figure 1) is a water-soluble, biodegradable and GRAS food antimicrobial compound active against bacteria, fungi, and yeast. It is a cationic polyamide naturally produced by the filamentous bacterium *Streptomyces albulus* with a variable number of L-lysine residues bound through amide linkage between ε-amino and α-carboxyl groups [34–36]. The antimicrobial activity comprises various mechanisms, such as intercellular reactions, changes in bacterial membrane permeability, interferences with the synthesis of bacterial cell protein and induction of the aggregation of bacterial proteins [36].

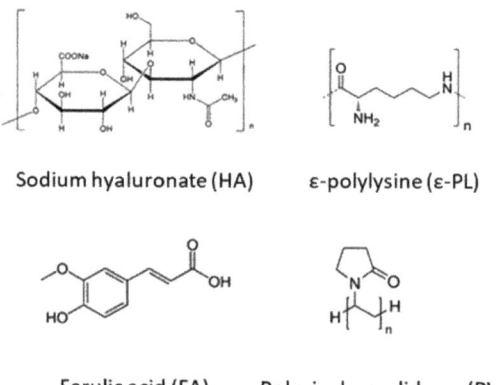

Figure 1. Chemical structures of polyvinyl pyrrolidone (PVP), hyaluronan (HA), ferulic acid (FA) and ε-polylysine (ε-PL).

The aim of this work was to design ocular inserts of HA-based fibers for ferulic acid (FA, Figure 1) and ε-PL dual delivery to the eye. FA has been recently the subject of intense research interest due to its wide range of therapeutic effects, including anti-oxidant properties, anti-aging, anti-inflammatory, neuroprotective and hematoprotective effects [37,38]. We hypothesized that FA combination with an antimicrobial peptide (ε-PL) could be used for the management of different ocular surface diseases. Due to its physico-chemical properties, HA has been chosen for designing electrospun nanofibers in attempt to modulate FA release to the ocular surface and protect it from light exposure. At first instance, preliminary design and characterization of HA based fibers was performed. Secondly, FA-loaded HA nanofibers were exposed to ε-PL for the simultaneous loading and crosslinking, and the obtained ocular inserts were evaluated in terms of microstructure, release patterns and antimicrobial activity.

2. Materials and Methods

2.1. Materials

Epsiliseen®-H (εPL, ε-polylysine, MW 4.7 kDa, Food Grade) was purchased from Siveele B.V. (Breda, Netherlands). Trans-ferulic acid (FA, MW 194.18 Da), Pluronic®F68 (poloxamer 188, PF68, MW 8.4 kDa), polyvinylpyrrolidone (PVP, MW 360 kDa), sodium hyaluronate (HA, MW 600–1100 kDa) and Tryptan blue powder were from Sigma Aldrich (St. Louis, MO, USA). Polyethylene oxide (PEO, MW 200 kDa) was purchased from Thermo Fisher Scientific (Waltham, MA, US). Ethanol absolute AnalaR Normapur®(EtOH, Reagent Ph Eur, Reagent USP) was purchased from VWR Chemicals (Milano, Italia). Water was purified using reverse osmosis (resistivity > 18 MΩ cm, MilliQ, Millipore®, Madrid, Spain). Supragradient HPLC grade acetonitrile and acetic acid glacial (reagent grade) were from Scharlau Chemicals (Barcelona, Spain). NaCl was from Panreac Quimica S.L.U. (Barcelona, Spain).

2.2. Nanofibers Preparation and Characterization

2.2.1. Polymer Dispersions

PVP was dissolved in EtOH:water 4:6 (v/v) mixture overnight under gentle magnetic stirring at room temperature at different concentrations (2.5%, 5%, 10% and 20% w/v). HA was then added to PVP solutions and hydrated under magnetic stirring overnight at room temperature; 20%, 10%, 5% and 2.5% w/v of HA were added to 20%, 10%, 5% and 2.5% w/v PVP solutions, respectively. The pH of the solutions was close to neutrality.

For FA-loaded nanofibers, the antioxidant was solubilized in a concentration equal to 0.5% w/v in EtOH:water 4:6 mixture (v/v) by vortexing before addition of PVP (5% w/v) and HA (0.8% w/v).

2.2.2. Rheology Analysis

Rheological analysis of electrospinning dispersions was performed using a Rheolyst AR-1000N rheometer fitted with an AR2500 data analyzer, a Peltier plate, and a 6-cm in diameter and 2.1° cone geometry (TA Instruments, Newcastle, UK). Viscosity measurements were recorded at 20 °C. Experiments were performed using a single batch for each dispersion.

2.2.3. Electrospinning Process

Solutions (5 mL) were electrospun onto an aluminum grounded target placed at 25 cm from the needle tip. The solutions were placed in a 5 mL plastic syringe of polypropylene connected to a 22-needle gauge (0.7 mm OD × 0.4 mm ID, Aldrich Chemical Co., Saint Louis, MO, USA). The flow rate and high-voltage power source were controlled using a Yflow®Professional Electrospinning Machine (Yflow®S.D., Malaga, Spain). Flow rates were 0.1 mL/h for PVP 2.5%–HA 1% and PVP 5%–HA 0.8% dispersions, 0.5 mL/h for PVP 10%–HA 0.5%, and 0.6 mL/h for PVP 20%–HA 0.2% dispersions. In absence of HA, flow rate of 1 mL/h was used for electrospinning 20% w/v PVP solution. Voltages applied to each solution were 15 kV for solutions containing 5%–20% w/v PVP, 18 kV for 2.5% w/v PVP solution and 25 kV for 10% w/v PVP solution (solely or mixed with HA). FA-loaded nanofibers were prepared from FA dispersion (0.5% FA, 5% PVP and 0.8% HA w/v) using 0.1 mL/h flow rate and 15 kV voltage. Electrospun fibers were deposited on a piece of aluminum foil above the aluminum collector plate. All experiments were carried out at room temperature and relative humidity of 30%–40%.

2.2.4. Quantification of FA Loading

Approx. 2 mg of FA-loaded nanofibers were immersed in 1 mL of MilliQ water for 5 min. Then, solutions were 20-fold diluted in MilliQ water and the absorbance recorded at 290 nm (UH5300

UV-Visible Spectrophotometer Hitachi, Chiyoda, Japan) for drug quantification. The experiments were carried out in triplicate.

2.2.5. Nanofibers Morphology

Scanning electron microscope (SEM) images of blank and drug-loaded nanofibers were obtained using a FESEM Ultra Plus (Zeiss, Oberkochen, Germany) at various magnifications. Samples were put onto metal plates and sputter-coated with 10 nm thick iridium film (Q150T-S, Quorum Technologies, Lewes, UK) before viewing.

2.3. Cross-Linked Inserts

2.3.1. Nanofibers Crosslinking

Nanofibers-based inserts were prepared by crosslinking with ε-PL. Nanofibers (10 ± 0.5 mg, area ≈ 2 cm^2, layer thickness ≈ 0.5 mm) were placed on a Petri dish and 0.05 mL ε-PL 50 mg/mL were poured onto the nanofibers. Mixtures were then casted and dried at 37 °C overnight.

2.3.2. Physical Characterization

Inserts thickness was measured using a Caliper Digital Electronic (Fowler™, Newton, MA, USA) and the weight recorded. SEM images of blank and FA-loaded inserts were obtained as described in Section 2.2.5.

2.3.3. FA Release

Blank and FA-loaded inserts (approx. 2.5 mg, 9-mm in diameter disks) were placed in wells containing 2 mL of NaCl 0.9% *w/v* of a 6 well plate at 35 °C under oscillation (100 osc/min, VWR®Incubating Mini Shaker, Spain). Release medium (1 mL) was sampled every 10 min and immediately replaced with the same volume of NaCl 0.9%. FA and ε-PL amounts released were monitored up to 30 min, and samples filtered before drug quantification (0.2 μm hydrophilic PTFE filters, Scharlab S.L., Barcelona, Spain).

FA was quantified using a reverse-phase Symmetry®C18 cartridge (3.9 × 150 mm, 5 μm, Waters, Milford, MA, USA), thermostated at 30 °C using a HPLC-UV system (Jasco LC Net II/ADC, SpectraLab Scientific Inc., Canada). The mobile phase was a mixture of acetonitrile: 2% acetic acid aqueous solution 19:81 (*v/v*) ratio, pumped at 1 mL/min. The injection volume was 90 μL and the absorbance was recorded at 290 nm. Retention time was 4.7 min. FA calibration curves were built in the range 5–25 μg/mL (R^2 > 0.999).

ε-PL quantification was performed by using a colorimetric method [39]. Briefly, Tryptan Blue aqueous solution (1 mg/mL, 25 μL) was added to ε-PL standard solutions or release samples (625 μL), and the mixtures incubated at 37 °C for 1 h. Mixtures were then centrifuged at 25 °C for 20 min at 8000 rpm. Finally, supernatants were analyzed at 589 nm (UH5300 UV-Visible Spectrophotometer, Hitachi, Chiyoda, Japan). ε-PL calibration curves were built in the range 0.5–10 μg/mL (R^2 > 0.992).

2.4. Biocompatibility and in vitro Antibacterial Activity Assessment

2.4.1. HET-CAM Test

Hen's Egg Test Chorioallantoic Membrane (HET-CAM) assay [40] was carried out using fertilized egg (50–60 g; Coren, Spain) previously incubated at 37 °C and 60% relative humidity (climatic chamber) for 9 days. The eggs were turned 3 times per day. The last day they were placed with the wider extreme upward for 12 h and then the eggshell was partially removed (2 cm in diameter) on the air chamber using a rotary saw (Dremel 300, Breda, Netherlands). The inner membrane was wet with 0.9% NaCl for 30 min in the climatic chamber and carefully removed. Pieces of 9-mm inserts were individually placed on the CAM of different eggs. Negative and positive controls were 0.9% NaCl and 0.1 M NaOH solutions, respectively. Photographs of CAM vessels were taken with a digital camera (Canon SX 260HS, without zoom) 5 min after the beginning of the assay and downloaded in the computer in JPEG format. GIMP®software was used to obtain a representative zone of the membrane with the tested formulations.

2.4.2. Fibroblast Compatibility

Fibers and inserts were weighed (4 mg) and added in separate to 1 mL of culture medium. The tubes were vortexed until specimen dissolution and kept at 37 °C. BalB/3T3 cells (CCL-163; ATCC, USA) were cultured at 37 °C in 75 cm^2 flasks using complete culture medium (DMEM supplemented with 10% v/v fetal bovine serum and 1% v/v penicillin/streptomycin/fungizone (PSF)) until 80% confluence was reached. Then, cells were trypsinized using TripLE solution (Sigma-Aldrich, MO, USA) and seeded in wells of 96 well plates (5000 cells/well). After 24 h, culture medium was removed and 100 µL of the sample solutions (4 mg/mL) and 100 µL of fresh culture medium were added to each well. Culture medium was used as negative control. Cells were again incubated at 37 °C for 24 or 48 h. At each timepoint, the medium was discarded and the cells were washed with PBS. Immediately after, freshly prepared CCK8 working solution (100 µL) consisting of 90 µL of culture medium and 10 µL of CCK-8 reagent (Sigma-Aldrich, MO, USA) was added to each well and then the cells incubated for 2 h at 37 °C. Finally, absorbance (450 nm) was recorded using a microplate reader (Model 8; BioRad, CA, USA).

2.4.3. Antibacterial Activity

The antibacterial activity was evaluated on Müller–Hinton agar plates seeded with *Pseudomonas aeruginosa* (CEC T110; $3.4 \cdot 10^9$ CFU/mL) or *Streptococcus aureus* (ATCC 25923; $1.2 \cdot 10^9$ CFU/mL). Blank and FA-loaded inserts were placed on the inoculated agar plates and the zones of inhibition were measured after incubation at 35 °C for 24 h. All experiments were carried out in duplicate.

2.5. Statistical Analysis

All data are reported as mean value ± sd. Differences were analyzed using ANOVA and multiple range test (Statgraphics Centurion XVI 1.15, StatPoint Technologies Inc., Warrenton, VA, USA). Differences were considered statistically significant when $p < 0.05$.

3. Results and Discussion

The present study was aimed at designing an ophthalmic platform able to increase FA residence time on the ocular surface, assuring in the meantime ε-PL release to the eye. Ophthalmic inserts could offer an increased ocular residence, controlled drug release and accurate dosing. The improved residence time of the drug in the conjunctival sac may enhance drug ocular availability with less frequent administration and fewer side effects than eyedrops [41].

3.1. HA Based Nanofibers

HA based nanofibrous membranes have been previously investigated as biomimetic tissue engineering scaffolds, wound healing materials, and drug delivery systems [42]. However, electrospinning of pure HA for scaffold preparation has been largely unsuccessful due to its inadequate physicochemical properties [29]. Indeed, high viscosity and surface tension hinder the electrospinning process and favor the fusion of electrospun nanofibers due to slow evaporation of the solvent [42]. It has been also reported that chain conformation of HA should change from the rigid alpha helix structure to the coil conformation for a successful electrospinning process [43]. Commonly, electrospinning requires polymers of quite high molecular weight and at a concentration above the critical overlapping value to facilitate chain entanglement in the dispersion and thus fiber formation during the electrical field-reduced flow [44]. Nevertheless, if polymer solution concentration is very high, bead fibers with thick diameters are formed because of the short drying time [45].

High MW sodium hyaluronan (MW 600–1100 kDa) was chosen for preparing electrospinning solutions at low concentrations. Preliminarily, electrospinning of HA aqueous dispersion was investigated. In accordance to literature [42], fibers solely were not obtained because of the instability of the jet (liquid atomization process, namely electrospraying). Thus, a small percentage of EtOH was added during the preparation of HA solutions to reduce the time needed for the solvent evaporation during electrospinning process. However, the addition of EtOH up to 20% *v/v* during the preparation of HA solutions (0.1%, 0.05% and 0.02% *w/v*) did not ameliorate the electrospinning process and the Taylor cone was not stable.

Incorporation of other chemical compounds was also investigated to overcome unfavorable physicochemical properties of HA solutions. Ionic surfactants may increase the net charge density and the instability of the charged jet leading to finer fibers [10]. The addition of 5% *w/v* Pluronic F68 to 0.2% *w/v* HA in 20% EtOH: 80% water and 40% EtOH: 60% water mixtures (*v/v*) did not lead to stable Taylor cone either. Similar results were observed by using 0.5% *w/v* HA concentration under the same conditions. The addition of PEO 200 (12% *w/v*) to 0.2%, 0.3%, 0.5%, 0.8% *w/v* HA aqueous solution did not improve the process either.

Next attempt was carried out with high molecular weight PVP (360 kDa) due to its already demonstrated capability to render electrospun nanofibers [33]. HA:PVP ratio and electrospinning parameters were adjusted to obtain a stable Taylor cone and consequently bead-free fibers with a sub-micron diameter. Particularly, various polymers concentrations were tested as fibers diameters could be highly dependent on this parameter and dispersion viscosity [5].

SEM micrographs of electrospun fibers prepared varying PVP and HA concentrations in EtOH:water 4:6 *v/v* are shown in Figure 2. Particles were detected in the case of PVP 2.5%–HA 1% *w/v* dispersions (not shown). Fibers with diameters of approx. 100 nm were obtained for 5% and 10% *w/v* PVP concentration; namely PVP 5%–HA 0.8% *w/v* and PVP 10%–HA 0.5% *w/v* had average diameters of 116 ± 48 and 48 ± 13 nm. An increase in PVP concentration to 20% *w/v* in both presence and absence of HA rendered fibers of approx. 1 μm; namely, the average diameters of PVP 20% *w/v* and PVP 20%–HA 0.2% *w/v* were 1224 ± 429 and 1166 ± 346 nm. The fibers showed homogenous surface indicating that all the process parameters were well controlled.

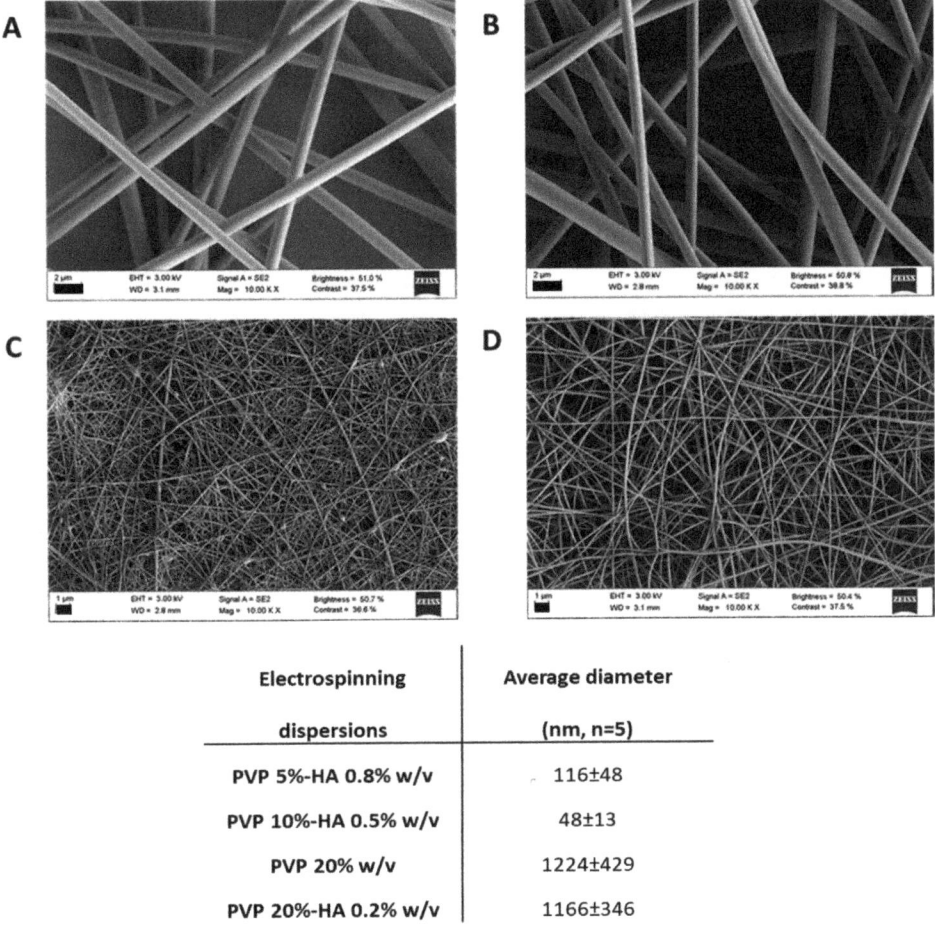

Electrospinning dispersions	Average diameter (nm, n=5)
PVP 5%-HA 0.8% w/v	116±48
PVP 10%-HA 0.5% w/v	48±13
PVP 20% w/v	1224±429
PVP 20%-HA 0.2% w/v	1166±346

Figure 2. SEM micrographs of PVP-HA nanofibers electrospun at 10 kV (A; PVP 20%, B; PVP 20%–HA 0.2%, C; PVP 10%–HA 0.5%, D; PVP 5%–HA 0.8%, scale bars 2 μm for A-B and 1 μm for C-D).

The high increase in fiber average diameter observed for PVP 20% *w/v* and PVP 20%–HA 0.2% *w/v* (Figure 2) is explained by the increase in viscosity (Figure 3) [32]. For drug loading, PVP 5%-HA 0.8% *w/v* dispersion was selected due to the sub-micron diameters of the obtained fibers and beads absence.

SEM of blank and FA-loaded nanofibers were comparable in morphology, demonstrating that FA incorporation did not have an impact on fiber morphology (Figure 4) and diameter (120 ± 26 nm). Additionally, the content in FA of the nanofibers was checked after electrospinning process (83.3 ± 14.0 μg/mg of fiber vs. theoretical 80 μg/mg of fiber) and confirmed that the application of high voltage field did not cause FA degradation.

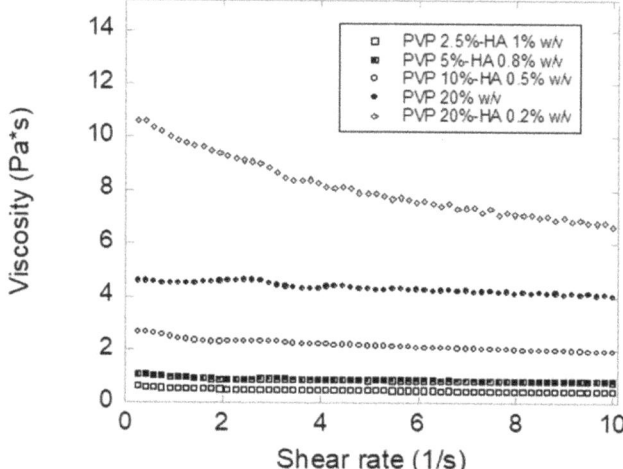

Figure 3. Viscosity measurements of electrospinning dispersions recorded at 20 °C.

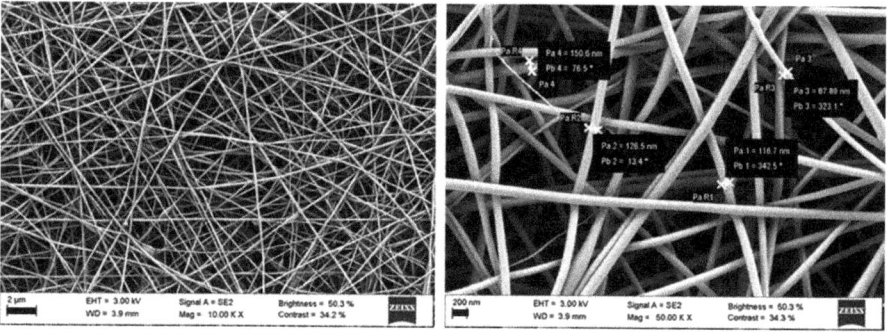

Figure 4. SEM of FA-loaded nanofibers obtained by electrospinning 0.5% FA, 5% PVP and 0.8% HA *w/v* dispersion (scale bars 2 μm on the left and 200 nm on the right).

3.2. Ocular Inserts of Nanofibers Crosslinked with ε-polylysine

Further studies were carried out with PVP 5%–HA 0.8% *w/v* nanofibers which were crosslinked with ε-PL taking benefit of the electrostatic interactions among the two polymers. Indeed, ε-PL is able to interact by electrostatic interactions with anionic polymers, and HA and ε-PL interactions have been already exploited for obtaining polyelectrolyte multilayers [46–48]. Apart from layer-by-layer structures, ε-PL is expected to interact with hyaluronan thanks to inter- and intra- molecular linkages between ε-PL amino groups and hyaluronan carboxylic groups forming macro-, micro- or nanohydrogels. In this study, electrostatic interactions were used to favor the crosslinking bonds between HA nanofibers to obtain inserts to be placed in the conjunctival sac.

Different mass ratios were tested by varying the concentration and the volume of the ε-PL solution to be added to HA nanofibers. As both PVP and HA are highly hydrophilic polymers, high concentration and small volume of the ε-PL solution to be added was selected (Fiber/ε-PL mass ratio equal to 2.4).

After crosslinking blank nanofibers, inserts appeared white with a mean thickness of 270 ± 21 μm and a weight of 39.5 ± 11.2 μg/cm^2. Conversely, crosslinked FA-loaded inserts appeared light yellow showing a mean thickness of 273 ± 41 μm and a weight of 46.8 ± 8.8 μg/cm^2. SEM images of blank cross-linked inserts revealed the presence of nanofibers structures even after electrostatic crosslinking, whereas these structures seemed not to be conserved on inserts surface in case of FA- loaded inserts (Figure 5) presumably due to electrostatic interactions between FA and the cross-linker ε-PL.

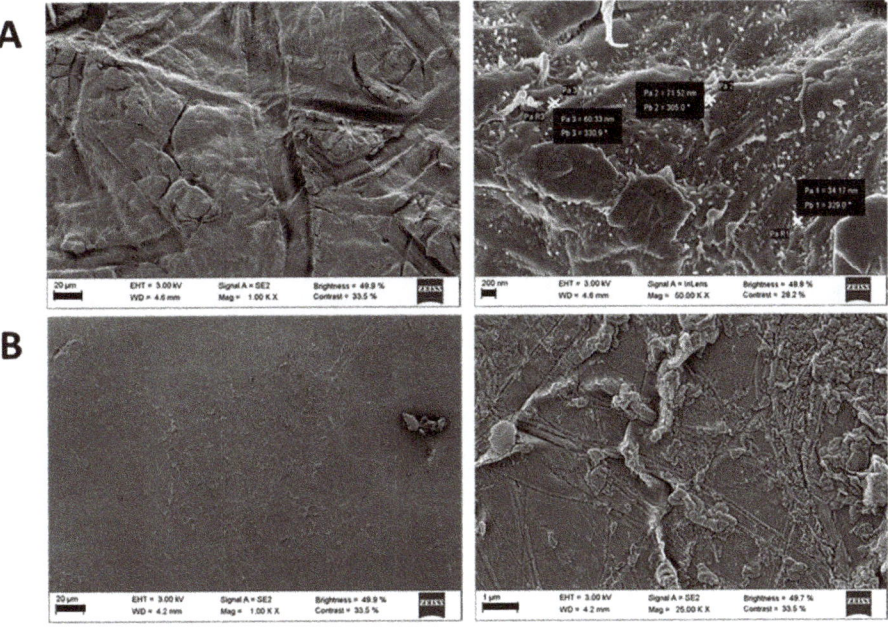

Figure 5. SEM micrographs of blank (**A**) and ferulic acid loaded (**B**) inserts (scale bars 20 μm on the left, 200 nm on the right at the top and 1 μm on the right at the bottom).

First screening of the ocular compatibility of the inserts with ocular tissues was assessed by HET-CAM assays. The chorioallantoic membrane of an embryonated hen's egg resembles the vascular conjunctiva of the eye. Thus, irritating effects after conjunctiva exposure of inserts can be predicted from changes in the chorioallantoic membrane [49]. In our case, none insert caused haemorrhage, vessels lysis or coagulation, and performed the same as the saline solution control (Figure 6). Adverse events occurred only in case of the positive control (NaOH 5 M), resulting in a rosette-like coagulation. Overall, HET-CAM results indicated that the designed inserts can be considered as non-irritant. These results were confirmed with a cytocompatibility study carried out with fibroblasts, which revealed cell viability values above 80% after 24 and 48 h in contact with blank and FA-loaded fibers and inserts.

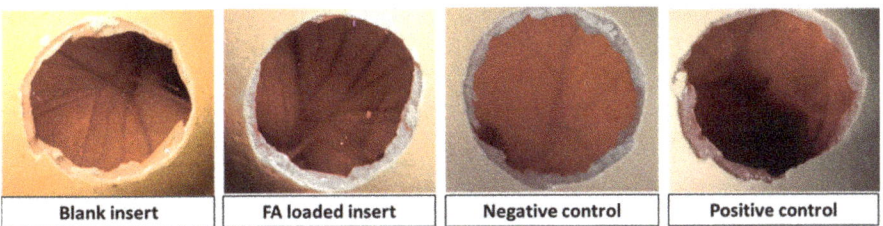

Figure 6. HET-CAM photographs after 5 min from the beginning of the test with blank and ferulic loaded inserts, and negative (0.9% NaCl solution) and positive (0.1 N NaOH solution) controls.

Then, the inserts were tested regarding their capability to release both FA and ε-PL. Although no specific methods are reported in Pharmacopoeias for studying drug release from ophthalmic dosage forms, in vitro studies under sink conditions in NaCl 0.9% medium may be useful as first step for studying the behavior of ophthalmic drug delivery systems [50]. The weight of the inserts was adjusted to have the same amount of FA and ε-PL. Blank and FA-loaded inserts eroded upon contact with saline solution in a short time interval (under the oscillation conditions tested) without noticeable swelling, and thus FA was released completely in 20 min. As shown in Figure 7, FA-loaded inserts (loading equal to 5.7% ± 0.2% *w/w*) released 91% ± 6% in 10 min and 100% of the loaded drug in 20 min. Concerning ε-PL loading, FA presence did not affect the peptide concentration into the inserts (12.2% ± 2.8% and 17.6% ± 3.1% w/w for blank and FA-loaded inserts) neither the peptide release. Blank inserts released 78% ± 20%, 77% ± 15% and 100% of ε-PL in 10, 20 and 30 min, respectively. Similarly, FA-loaded inserts released 70% ± 26%, 93% ± 9% and 100% of peptide in 10, 20 and 30 min, respectively. It should be noticed that under physiological conditions the volume of tears is limited and thus the insert could hydrate, adhere to the mucus on the ocular surface and release the drug more slowly [51,52]. Strong antioxidant activity of FA has been reported for concentrations of 1 mg/mL [53], which could be provided by the inserts (0.14 mg FA in the 2.5 mg insert) on the ocular surface in few minutes after application.

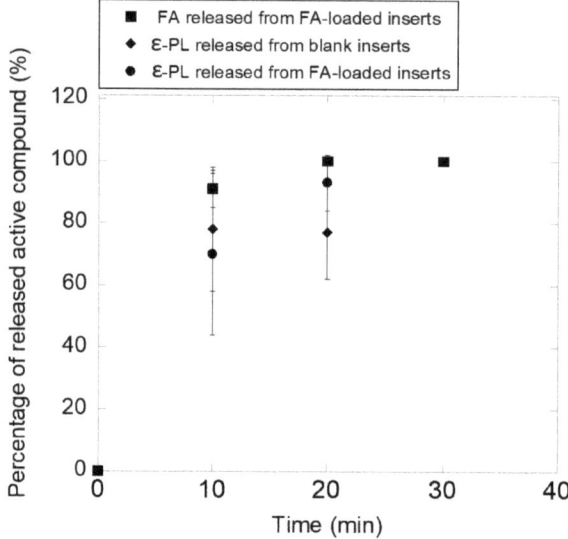

Figure 7. FA and ε-PL release patterns from blank and FA loaded inserts (mean ± sd, n = 3).

Lastly, blank and FA-loaded inserts were challenged against *Pseudomonas aeruginosa* and *Staphylococcus aureus* and the growth inhibition zones (Figure 8) were measured after 24 h of incubation. Differently to the starting fibers which did not show any antimicrobial activity (data not shown), blank and FA-loaded inserts resulted effective against both microbial species. This antibacterial efficacy can be ascribed to the presence of the peptide into the inserts. Indeed, the antibacterial mechanism of ε-PL against Gram-positive and Gram-negative bacteria has been attributed to membrane disruption related to the interactions of the primary amine surface groups with the cell membrane [54,55]. However, a solution prepared with the PL concentration expected to be provided by the inserts did not cause growth inhibition. Although the reasons for this finding are not clear, they may be related to the fact that the insert retains PL on its surface while the solution may freely diffuse to the agar medium and become diluted and thus inefficient.

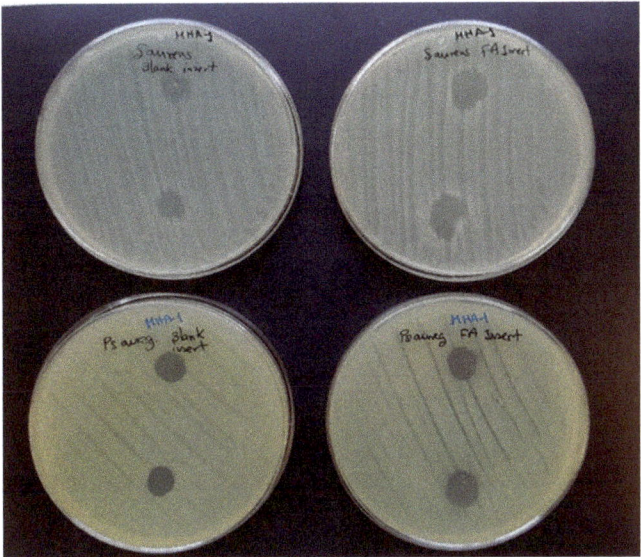

Figure 8. *Staphylococcus aureus* (first row) and *Pseudomonas aeruginosa* (second row) inhibition zones caused by blank and FA-loaded inserts.

4. Conclusions

HA nanofibers were successfully obtained in presence of PVP, showing proper dimensions and ferulic acid loading. Crosslinked inserts were obtained by crosslinking nanofibers with ε-PL and evaluated for a possible ocular application. Crosslinked inserts showed adequate thickness, release pattern, in vitro biocompatibility and antibacterial activity. Further ex vivo and in vivo studies (in particular, the permanence time of the formulation on sclera/conjunctiva and FA permeability) may contribute to forecast the suitability of the crosslinked inserts for ocular application.

Author Contributions: Conceptualization, M.A.G. and C.A.-L.; methodology, M.A.G.; validation, M.A.G. and C.A.-L.; resources, M.A.G.; data curation, C.A.-L.; writing—Original draft preparation, M.A.G.; writing—Review and editing, M.A.G. and C.A.-L.; supervision, A.C.; project administration, C.A.-L. and A.C.; funding acquisition, C.A.-L. and A.C. All authors have read and agreed to the published version of the manuscript.

Funding: This research was funded by the Spanish MINECO (grant number SAF2017-83118-R), Agencia Estatal de Investigación (AEI) Spain, Xunta de Galicia (grant numbers ED431C 2016/008 and AEMAT ED431E 2018/08), and FEDER.

Conflicts of Interest: The authors declare no conflict of interest.

References

1. Bhattarai, R.S.; Bachu, R.D.; Boddu, S.H.S.; Bhaduri, S. Biomedical Applications of Electrospun Nanofibers: Drug and Nanoparticle Delivery. *Pharmaceutics* **2018**, *11*, 5. [CrossRef]
2. Shahriar, S.M.S.; Mondal, J.; Hasan, M.N.; Revuri, V.; Lee, D.Y.; Lee, Y.K. Electrospinning Nanofibers for Therapeutics Delivery. *Nanomaterials* **2019**, *9*, 532. [CrossRef]
3. Afshari, M. 1—Introduction. In *Electrospun Nanofibers*; Afshari, M., Ed.; Woodhead Publishing: Sawston/Cambridge, UK, 2017; pp. 1–8.
4. Salas, C. 4—Solution electrospinning of nanofibers. In *Electrospun Nanofibers*; Afshari, M., Ed.; Woodhead Publishing: Sawston/Cambridge, UK, 2017; pp. 73–108.
5. Pelipenko, J.; Kocbek, P.; Kristl, J. Critical attributes of nanofibers: Preparation, drug loading, and tissue regeneration. *Int. J. Pharm.* **2015**, *484*, 57–74. [CrossRef]

6. Jang, J.H.; Castano, O.; Kim, H.W. Electrospun materials as potential platforms for bone tissue engineering. *Adv. Drug Deliv. Rev.* **2009**, *61*, 1065–1083. [CrossRef]
7. Xie, J.; Li, X.; Lipner, J.; Manning, C.N.; Schwartz, A.G.; Thomopoulos, S.; Xia, Y. "Aligned-to-random" nanofiber scaffolds for mimicking the structure of the tendon-to-bone insertion site. *Nanoscale* **2010**, *2*, 923–926. [CrossRef] [PubMed]
8. Zhang, X.; Thomas, V.; Xu, Y.; Bellis, S.L.; Vohra, Y.K. An in vitro regenerated functional human endothelium on a nanofibrous electrospun scaffold. *Biomaterials* **2010**, *31*, 4376–4381. [CrossRef] [PubMed]
9. Zeng, J.; Xu, X.; Chen, X.; Liang, Q.; Bian, X.; Yang, L.; Jing, X. Biodegradable electrospun fibers for drug delivery. *J. Control. Release* **2003**, *92*, 227–231. [CrossRef]
10. Salas, C.; Thompson, Z.; Bhattarai, N. 15—Electrospun chitosan fibers. In *Electrospun Nanofibers*; Afshari, M., Ed.; Woodhead Publishing: Sawston/Cambridge, UK, 2017; pp. 371–398.
11. Sebe, I.; Szabó, P.; Kállai-Szabó, B.; Zelkó, R. Incorporating small molecules or biologics into nanofibers for optimized drug release: A review. *Int. J. Pharm.* **2015**, *494*, 516–530. [CrossRef]
12. Sun, X.; Yu, Z.; Cai, Z.; Yu, L.; Lv, Y. Voriconazole Composited Polyvinyl Alcohol/Hydroxypropyl-beta-Cyclodextrin Nanofibers for Ophthalmic Delivery. *PLoS ONE* **2016**, *11*, e0167961. [CrossRef]
13. Da Silva, G.R.; Lima, T.H.; Fernandes-Cunha, G.M.; Oréfice, R.L.; Da Silva-Cunha, A.; Zhao, M.; Behar-Cohen, F. Ocular biocompatibility of dexamethasone acetate loaded poly(ε-caprolactone) nanofibers. *Eur. J. Pharm. Biopharm.* **2019**, *142*, 20–30. [CrossRef]
14. Bhattarai, R.S.; Das, A.; Alzhrani, R.M.; Kang, D.; Bhaduri, S.B.; Boddu, S.H.S. Comparison of electrospun and solvent cast polylactic acid (PLA)/poly(vinyl alcohol) (PVA) inserts as potential ocular drug delivery vehicles. *Mater. Sci. Eng. C Mater. Biol. Appl.* **2017**, *77*, 895–903. [CrossRef] [PubMed]
15. Göttel, B.; de Souza e Silva, J.M.; Santos de Oliveira, C.; Syrowatka, F.; Fiorentzis, M.; Viestenz, A.; Viestenz, A.; Mäder, K. Electrospun nanofibers—A promising solid in-situ gelling alternative for ocular drug delivery. *Eur. J. Pharm. Biopharm.* **2020**, *146*, 125–132. [CrossRef] [PubMed]
16. Gaudana, R.; Ananthula, H.K.; Parenky, A.; Mitra, A.K. Ocular drug delivery. *AAPS J.* **2010**, *12*, 348–360. [CrossRef]
17. de Souza, S.O.L.; Guerra, M.C.A.; Heneine, L.G.D.; de Oliveira, C.R.; Cunha Junior, A.D.S.; Fialho, S.L.; Orefice, R.L. Biodegradable core-shell electrospun nanofibers containing bevacizumab to treat age-related macular degeneration. *J. Mater. Sci. Mater. Med.* **2018**, *29*, 173. [CrossRef] [PubMed]
18. Yellanki, S.K.; Anna, B.; Kishan, M.R. Preparation and in vivo evaluation of sodium alginate—Poly (vinyl alcohol) electrospun nanofibers of forskolin for glaucoma treatment. *Pak. J. Pharm. Sci.* **2019**, *32*, 669–674. [PubMed]
19. Karatas, A.; Algan, A.H.; Pekel-Bayramgil, N.; Turhan, F.; Altanlar, N. Ofloxacin Loaded Electrospun Fibers for Ocular Drug Delivery: Effect of Formulation Variables on Fiber Morphology and Drug Release. *Curr. Drug Deliv.* **2016**, *13*, 433–443. [CrossRef]
20. Lancina, M.G., 3rd; Singh, S.; Kompella, U.B.; Husain, S.; Yang, H. Fast Dissolving Dendrimer Nanofiber Mats as Alternative to Eye Drops for More Efficient Antiglaucoma Drug Delivery. *ACS Biomater. Sci. Eng.* **2017**, *3*, 1861–1868. [CrossRef]
21. Zhang, Z.; Yu, J.; Zhou, Y.; Zhang, R.; Song, Q.; Lei, L.; Li, X. Supramolecular nanofibers of dexamethasone derivatives to form hydrogel for topical ocular drug delivery. *Colloids Surf. B Biointerfaces* **2018**, *164*, 436–443. [CrossRef]
22. Cejkova, J.; Cejka, C.; Trosan, P.; Zajicova, A.; Sykova, E.; Holan, V. Treatment of alkali-injured cornea by cyclosporine A-loaded electrospun nanofibers—An alternative mode of therapy. *Exp. Eye Res.* **2016**, *147*, 128–137. [CrossRef]
23. Mirzaeei, S.; Berenjian, K.; Khazaei, R. Preparation of the Potential Ocular Inserts by Electrospinning Method to Achieve the Prolong Release Profile of Triamcinolone Acetonide. *Adv. Pharm. Bull.* **2018**, *8*, 21–27. [CrossRef]
24. Singla, J.; Bajaj, T.; Goyal, A.K.; Rath, G. Development of Nanofibrous Ocular Insert for Retinal Delivery of Fluocinolone Acetonide. *Curr. Eye Res.* **2019**, *44*, 541–550. [CrossRef] [PubMed]
25. Khalil, I.; Ali, I.; El-Sherbiny, I. Noninvasive biodegradable nanoparticles-in-nanofibers single-dose ocular insert: In vitro, ex vivo and in vivo evaluation. *Nanomedicine* **2018**, *14*, 33—55. [CrossRef] [PubMed]

26. Oldenkamp, H.F.; Vela Ramirez, J.E.; Peppas, N.A. Re-evaluating the importance of carbohydrates as regenerative biomaterials. *Regen. Biomater.* **2019**, *6*, 1–12. [CrossRef] [PubMed]
27. Seon-Lutz, M.; Couffin, A.C.; Vignoud, S.; Schlatter, G.; Hebraud, A. Electrospinning in water and in situ crosslinking of hyaluronic acid/cyclodextrin nanofibers: Towards wound dressing with controlled drug release. *Carbohydr. Polym.* **2019**, *207*, 276–287. [CrossRef]
28. Petrova, V.A.; Chernyakov, D.D.; Poshina, D.N.; Gofman, I.V.; Romanov, D.P.; Mishanin, A.I.; Golovkin, A.S.; Skorik, Y.A. Electrospun Bilayer Chitosan/Hyaluronan Material and Its Compatibility with Mesenchymal Stem Cells. *Materials* **2019**, *12*, 2016. [CrossRef]
29. Chanda, A.; Adhikari, J.; Ghosh, A.; Chowdhury, S.R.; Thomas, S.; Datta, P.; Saha, P. Electrospun chitosan/polycaprolactone-hyaluronic acid bilayered scaffold for potential wound healing applications. *Int. J. Biol. Macromol.* **2018**, *116*, 774–785. [CrossRef]
30. Nair, B. Final Report On the Safety Assessment of Polyvinylpyrrolidone (PVP). *Int. J. Toxicol.* **1998**, *17*, 95–130. [CrossRef]
31. Aghamohamadi, N.; Sanjani, N.S.; Majidi, R.F.; Nasrollahi, S.A. Preparation and characterization of Aloe vera acetate and electrospinning fibers as promising antibacterial properties materials. *Mater. Sci. Eng. C Mater. Biol. Appl.* **2019**, *94*, 445–452. [CrossRef]
32. Costoya, A.; Ballarin, F.M.; Llovo, J.; Concheiro, A.; Abraham, G.A.; Alvarez-Lorenzo, C. HMDSO-plasma coated electrospun fibers of poly(cyclodextrin)s for antifungal dressings. *Int. J. Pharm.* **2016**, *513*, 518–527. [CrossRef]
33. Oryan, A.; Kamali, A.; Moshiri, A.; Baharvand, H.; Daemi, H. Chemical crosslinking of biopolymeric scaffolds: Current knowledge and future directions of crosslinked engineered bone scaffolds. *Int. J. Biol. Macromol.* **2018**, *107*, 678–688. [CrossRef]
34. Yoshida, T.; Nagasawa, T. epsilon-Poly-L-lysine: Microbial production, biodegradation and application potential. *Appl. Microbiol. Biotechnol.* **2003**, *62*, 21–26. [CrossRef] [PubMed]
35. Shih, I.L.; Shen, M.H.; Van, Y.T. Microbial synthesis of poly(epsilon-lysine) and its various applications. *Bioresour. Technol.* **2006**, *97*, 1148–1159. [CrossRef] [PubMed]
36. Shima, S.; Matsuoka, H.; Iwamoto, T.; Sakai, H. Antimicrobial action of epsilon-poly-L-lysine. *J. Antibiot.* **1984**, *37*, 1449–1455. [CrossRef] [PubMed]
37. Zdunska, K.; Dana, A.; Kolodziejczak, A.; Rotsztejn, H. Antioxidant Properties of Ferulic Acid and Its Possible Application. *Skin Pharmacol. Physiol.* **2018**, *31*, 332–336. [CrossRef]
38. Tsai, C.Y.; Woung, L.C.; Yen, J.C.; Tseng, P.C.; Chiou, S.H.; Sung, Y.J.; Liu, K.T.; Cheng, Y.H. Thermosensitive chitosan-based hydrogels for sustained release of ferulic acid on corneal wound healing. *Carbohydr. Polym.* **2016**, *135*, 308–315. [CrossRef]
39. Grotzky, A.; Manaka, Y.; Fornera, S.; Willeke, M.; Walde, P. Quantification of α-polylysine: A comparison of four UV/V is spectrophotometric methods. *Anal. Methods* **2010**, *2*, 1448–1455. [CrossRef]
40. Steiling, W.; Bracher, M.; Courtellemont, P.; de Silva, O. The HET-CAM, a Useful In Vitro Assay for Assessing the Eye Irritation Properties of Cosmetic Formulations and Ingredients. *Toxicol. In Vitro* **1999**, *13*, 375–384. [CrossRef]
41. Saettone, M.F.; Salminen, L. Ocular inserts for topical delivery. *Adv. Drug Deliv. Rev.* **1995**, *16*, 95–106. [CrossRef]
42. Lee, K.Y.; Jeong, L.; Kang, Y.O.; Lee, S.J.; Park, W.H. Electrospinning of polysaccharides for regenerative medicine. *Adv. Drug Deliv. Rev.* **2009**, *61*, 1020–1032. [CrossRef]
43. Liu, Y.; Ma, G.; Fang, D.; Xu, J.; Zhang, H.; Nie, J. Effects of solution properties and electric field on the electrospinning of hyaluronic acid. *Carbohydr. Polym.* **2011**, *83*, 1011–1015. [CrossRef]
44. Costoya, A.; Concheiro, A.; Alvarez-Lorenzo, C. Electrospun Fibers of Cyclodextrins and Poly(cyclodextrins). *Molecules* **2017**, *22*, 230. [CrossRef] [PubMed]
45. Khajavi, R.; Abbasipour, M. 5—Controlling nanofiber morphology by the electrospinning process. In *Electrospun Nanofibers*; Afshari, M., Ed.; Woodhead Publishing: Sawston/Cambridge, UK, 2017; pp. 109–123.
46. Niepel, M.S.; Ekambaram, B.K.; Schmelzer, C.E.H.; Groth, T. Polyelectrolyte multilayers of poly (l-lysine) and hyaluronic acid on nanostructured surfaces affect stem cell response. *Nanoscale* **2019**, *11*, 2878–2891. [CrossRef] [PubMed]

47. Prokopovic, V.Z.; Vikulina, A.S.; Sustr, D.; Shchukina, E.M.; Shchukin, D.G.; Volodkin, D.V. Binding Mechanism of the Model Charged Dye Carboxyfluorescein to Hyaluronan/Polylysine Multilayers. *ACS Appl. Mater. Interfaces* **2017**, *9*, 38908–38918. [CrossRef] [PubMed]
48. Dreaden, E.C.; Morton, S.W.; Shopsowitz, K.E.; Choi, J.H.; Deng, Z.J.; Cho, N.J.; Hammond, P.T. Bimodal tumor-targeting from microenvironment responsive hyaluronan layer-by-layer (LbL) nanoparticles. *ACS Nano* **2014**, *8*, 8374–8382. [CrossRef] [PubMed]
49. Kishore, A.S.; Surekha, P.A.; Sekhar, P.V.; Srinivas, A.; Murthy, P.B. Hen egg chorioallantoic membrane bioassay: An in vitro alternative to draize eye irritation test for pesticide screening. *Int. J. Toxicol.* **2008**, *27*, 449–453. [CrossRef] [PubMed]
50. Alvarez-Rivera, F.; Serro, A.P.; Silva, D.; Concheiro, A.; Alvarez-Lorenzo, C. Hydrogels for diabetic eyes: Naltrexone loading, release profiles and cornea penetration. *Mater. Sci. Eng. C* **2019**, *105*, 110092. [CrossRef] [PubMed]
51. Kumari, A.; Sharma, P.K.; Garg, V.K.; Garg, G. Ocular inserts—Advancement in therapy of eye diseases. *J. Adv. Pharm. Technol. Res.* **2010**, *1*, 291–296. [CrossRef]
52. Foureaux, G.; Franca, J.J.R.; Nogueira, C.; Fulgencio Gde, O.; Ribeiro, T.G.; Castilho, R.O.; Yoshida, M.I.; Fuscaldi, L.L.; Fernandes, S.O.; Cardoso, V.N.; et al. Ocular Inserts for Sustained Release of the Angiotensin-Converting Enzyme 2 Activator, Diminazene Aceturate, to Treat Glaucoma in Rats. *PLoS ONE* **2015**, *10*, e0133149. [CrossRef]
53. Grimaudo, M.A.; Amato, G.; Carbone, C.; Diaz-Rodriguez, P.; Musumeci, T.; Concheiro, A.; Alvarez-Lorenzo, C.; Puglisi, G. Micelle-nanogel platform for ferulic acid ocular delivery. *Int. J. Pharm.* **2020**, *576*, 118986. [CrossRef]
54. Ye, R.; Xu, H.; Wan, C.; Peng, S.; Wang, L.; Xu, H.; Aguilar, Z.P.; Xiong, Y.; Zeng, Z.; Wei, H. Antibacterial activity and mechanism of action of ε-poly-l-lysine. *Biochem. Biophys. Res. Commun.* **2013**, *439*, 148–153. [CrossRef]
55. Amariei, G.; Kokol, V.; Vivod, V.; Boltes, K.; Letón, P.; Rosal, R. Biocompatible antimicrobial electrospun nanofibers functionalized with ε-poly-l-lysine. *Int. J. Pharm.* **2018**, *553*, 141–148. [CrossRef] [PubMed]

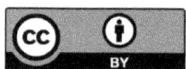

© 2020 by the authors. Licensee MDPI, Basel, Switzerland. This article is an open access article distributed under the terms and conditions of the Creative Commons Attribution (CC BY) license (http://creativecommons.org/licenses/by/4.0/).

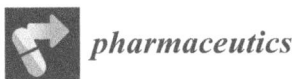

Article

Evaluation and Comparison of Solid Lipid Nanoparticles (SLNs) and Nanostructured Lipid Carriers (NLCs) as Vectors to Develop Hydrochlorothiazide Effective and Safe Pediatric Oral Liquid Formulations

Paola Mura [1], Francesca Maestrelli [1], Mario D'Ambrosio [2], Cristina Luceri [2] and Marzia Cirri [1,*]

[1] Department of Chemistry, University of Florence, via Schiff 6, Sesto Fiorentino, 50019 Florence, Italy; paola.mura@unifi.it (P.M.); francesca.maestrelli@unifi.it (F.M.)
[2] Department of Neurofarba, University of Florence, Viale Pieraccini 6, 50139 Florence, Italy; mario.dambrosio@unifi.it (M.D.); cristina.luceri@unifi.it (C.L.)
* Correspondence: marzia.cirri@unifi.it; Tel.: +39-055-4573674

Abstract: The aim of this study was the optimization of solid lipid nanoparticles (SLN) and nanostructured lipid carriers (NLC) in terms of physicochemical and biopharmaceutical properties, to develop effective and stable aqueous liquid formulations of hydrochlorothiazide, suitable for paediatric therapy, overcoming its low-solubility and poor-stability problems. Based on solubility studies, Precirol® ATO5 and Transcutol® HP were used as solid and liquid lipids, respectively. The effect of different surfactants, also in different combinations and at different amounts, on particle size, homogeneity and surface-charge of nanoparticles was carefully investigated. The best formulations were selected for drug loading, and evaluated also for entrapment efficiency and release behaviour. For both SLN and NLC series, the use of Gelucire® 44/14 as surfactant rather than PluronicF68 or Tween® 80 yielded a marked particle size reduction (95–75 nm compared to around 600–400 nm), and an improvement in entrapment efficiency and drug release rate. NLC showed a better performance than SLN, reaching about 90% entrapped drug (vs. 80%) and more than 90% drug released after 300 min (vs. about 65%). All selected formulations showed good physical stability during 6-month storage at 4 °C, but a higher loss of encapsulated drug was found for SLNs (15%) than for NLCs (<5%). Moreover, all selected formulations revealed the absence of any cytotoxic effect, as assessed by a cell-viability test on Caco-2 cells and are able to pass the intestinal epithelium as suggested by Caco-2 uptake experiments.

Keywords: solid lipid nanoparticles; nanostructured lipid carriers; hydrochlorothiazide; pediatric therapy; Gelucire; cytotoxicity; cellular uptake

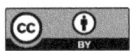

1. Introduction

Drugs belonging to the cardiovascular group are largely utilized in paediatric therapy, due to their several indications in severe and/or chronic clinical conditions such as heart failure, hypertension, hypovolemic shock or oedema. However, the European Medicines Agency (EMA) pointed out that a limited number of antihypertensive drugs is available in suitable formulation for paediatrics [1]. Among these, hydrochlorothiazide (HCT) is one of the diuretic drugs most widely used in the treatment of paediatric hypertension, being also present in the World Health Organization (WHO) Model List of Essential Medicines for Children [2]. This is due to the fact that diuretic drugs, and particularly HCT, have a long history of safety and therapeutic efficacy, based on clinical experience in hypertensive children, resulting appropriate for paediatric use [3]. Moreover, the HCT single daily administration makes it easier to be accepted by young patients, thus improving their compliance to the pharmacologic therapy [4].

However, HCT has been classified as a Class IV drug in the Biopharmaceutical Classification System (BCS) due to its poor solubility and low membrane permeability [5,6], often resulting in a low and variable oral availability [7]. Additionally, different studies [8–11] evidenced problems of stability of this drug in aqueous solutions. For all these reasons, no liquid formulations of HCT are currently present on the market. This gives rise to some limitations in its utilization in paediatrics, where the use of oral solid dosage forms is restricted by their rigid dose content and by the difficulty of children to swallow them [12]. On the other hand, the common practice of caregivers to prepare extemporaneous liquid formulations by crushing of tablets or capsules opening, and then suspending the powder in a suitable liquid, can often lead to loss of accuracy of the dosage, issues with stability, and possible errors due to incorrect manipulation [13,14]. Moreover, excipients present in dosage forms designed for adults could be harmful to children, particularly for neonates and infants [15,16]. Therefore, the development of a stable HCT liquid formulation suitable for paediatric use would allow to overcome all the above drawbacks and make its therapeutic use easier, safer and more effective.

Lipid-based nanocarriers emerged as a powerful approach to enhance the stability and oral bioavailability of poorly soluble drugs. Moreover, in virtue of their biocompatibility, biodegradability and absence of toxicity [17,18], they can be considered suitable also for pediatric formulations. Among these carriers, solid lipid nanoparticles (SLNs), formed by a dispersion of solid, biocompatible lipids in an aqueous phase, proved to be a valid alternative to liposomes, providing similar benefits in terms of safety in use, but overcoming some of their main disadvantages, such as the limited stability and poor entrapment efficiency [19,20]. Furthermore, the solid lipid matrix can offer a better protection of the entrapped drug [21]. An oral liquid pediatric formulation of HCT loaded in SLNs has recently been proposed, endowed with satisfactory encapsulation efficiency (near to 60%) and acceptable storage stability (1 month) [22].

Nanostructured lipid carriers (NLCs) represent another interesting type of lipid nanocarrier, planned with the purpose of improving some potential shortcomings presented by SLNs, especially their propensity to throw out the drug from the matrix during the storage, due to the highly ordered status of the crystalline solid lipid [23]. In fact, differently from SLNs, the solid matrix of NLCs is formed by a mixture of biocompatible solid and liquid lipids, thus giving rise to a less-ordered, imperfect structure, which should ensure improved physical stability, higher drug loading ability and lower tendency to prematurely leak the drug during storage [24]. Actually, a NLC-based oral liquid pediatric formulation of HCT recently developed proved to be more effective than the previous SLN drug formulation, both in terms of drug entrapment efficacy (around 90% vs. 60%) and storage stability (3 months vs. 1 month) [25].

Considering these interesting and promising results, it seemed worthy of interest to further investigate and compare the effectiveness of SLNs and NLCs as carriers for the development of suitable oral liquid pediatric formulations of HCT, by particularly focusing the attention on the proper choice of the most effective solid and liquid lipid components and carefully investigating the effect of different surfactants, also in combinations and at different amounts, in order to optimize the nanoparticle properties (in terms of size, homogeneity, entrapment efficiency and storage stability). Cytoxicity and cellular uptake studies were finally performed using Caco-2 cells, in order, respectively, to verify the safe use of the selected formulations, and to assess their ability to enter the intestinal epithelium cells.

2. Materials and Methods
2.1. Materials

Hydrochlorothiazide (HCT) was a generous gift of Menarini (Florence, Italy). Glyceryl distearate/palmitostearate (Precirol® ATO5), high-purity diethylene glycol monoethyl ether (Transcutol P), highest-purity diethylene glycol monoethyl ether (Transcutol® HP), glyceryl dibehenate (Compritol® 888 ATO), lauroylpolyoxyl-32-glycerides (Gelucire® 44/14), glyceryl monostearate 40/55 (Type I) (Geleol®), cetyl palmitate, caprylic/capric triglycerides (Labrafac® Lipophile WL 1349), PEG-8-caprylic/capric glycerides (Labrasol®) and caprylocaproyl polyoxyl-8 glycerides (Labrasol ALF), were kindly provided by Gattefossé (Cedex, France). Glyceryl tripalmitate (Tripalmitin) and Rhodamine 6G were from Sigma Aldrich (St. Louis, MO, USA), glyceryl monostearate (Imwitor® 491) and medium chain (C8-C10) triglycerides (Miglyol® 810N) were kindly provided by Cremer Oleo GmbH (Witten, Germany). Caprylic triglycerides (Miglyol® 812) was from Sasol GmbH (Witten, Germany), polyoxyethylen-sorbitan monoleate (Tween® 80) from Merck (Hohenbrunn, Germany) and poloxamer 188 (Pluronic® F68) from BASF (Ludwigshafen, Germany). Purified water was obtained by reverse osmosis (Elix 3 Millipore, Rockville, MD, USA). All other chemicals were of reagent grade and used as received.

2.2. Screening of Solid and Liquid Lipids
2.2.1. Solubilizing Power of Solid and Liquid Lipids towards the Drug

HCT solubility in different solid and liquid lipids was assessed, in order to select the most effective ones for SLN and NLC preparation.

The solubility in solid lipids was determined by adding 100 mg of HCT to 5 g of the lipid and then heating the obtained mixture until the lipid melted; the drug solubility in the melt lipid was visually estimated by establishing the achievement of a clear solution and the absence of drug crystals [26].

The solubility in liquid lipids was instead determined by adding 100 mg of HCT to 5 mL of liquid lipid and allowing to reach equilibrium (24 h) at 65 °C (to mimic the temperature conditions used during NLC preparation); the drug solubility was then evaluated by visual checking of dissolution of HCT crystals and obtainment of a perfectly transparent, homogeneous system [27].

2.2.2. Compatibility Studies by Differential Scanning Calorimetry (DSC)

Compatibility studies were performed by Differential Scanning Calorimetry (DSC) with a Mettler TA4000 (Star^e Software) apparatus (Mettler Toledo, Switzerland) equipped with a DSC 25 cell. Samples were accurately weighed (Mettler M3 microbalance) and scanned in pierced Al pans under static air (10 °C/min, 30–300 °C). Indium was used as a standard (99.98% purity; T_{fus}: 156.61 °C; ΔH_{fus}: 28.71 J/g) for temperature and heat flow calibration. Pure drug and components of SLN or NLC and their different combinations at the same ratio used in the final formulation were analysed.

2.3. Preparation of Lipid Nanoparticles

SLNs and NLCs were prepared using the Hot High-Shear Homogenization (HSH) technique followed by ultrasonication as described by Cirri et al., 2018 [25]. Briefly, in the case of SLNs, empty nanoparticles were prepared by heating at 65 °C, up to melting the selected solid lipid (5 g). In the meanwhile, the aqueous phase, containing the surfactant (Gelucire® 44/14, Tween® 80, Pluronic® F68, at different %, separately or in mixtures) was heated at the same temperature and then 10 mL were dispersed in the fused lipid by 5 or 10 min homogenization at 10,000 rpm (high shear homogenizer Silverson L5M, Chesham, UK). The pre-emulsion was then subjected to 3 min sonication (amplitude 50%, power 100 W) (Sonopuls HD 2200 sonicator, Bandelin Electronics, Berlin, Germany). The obtained dispersion was finally cooled down to 4 °C.

The procedure for NLCs production was the same, but a liquid lipid was initially added to the solid one at different percentages (0.5, 1, 3 and 5%) and then heated together.

In the case of nanoparticles loaded with HCT, the drug was in all cases added to the lipid phase, so that to have a final concentration of 0.2% w/v.

All formulations were stored at 4 °C for further investigations.

2.4. Characterization of Lipid Nanoparticles (NPs)

2.4.1. Measurement of Particle Size, Polydispersity Index and ζ (Zeta) Potential

Mean diameter and polydispersity index (PDI) of nanoparticles were determined at 25 °C by dynamic light scattering (DLS) using a Zetasizer Nano ZS (Malvern Instruments Ltd., Malvern, UK). Zeta potential (ZP) of nanoparticles was measured by laser Doppler micro-electrophoresis using a Zetasizer Nano ZS (Malvern Instruments Ltd., Malvern, UK). Before measurements, all samples were diluted appropriately with purified water. All analyses were carried out on three samples for each formulation, and the mean value was calculated for each measured parameter.

2.4.2. Determination of Entrapment Efficiency (EE%)

Drug entrapment efficiency was determined by an indirect method, according to Cirri et al., 2012 [28], after separation of the unincorporated drug from drug-loaded nanoparticles by ultrafiltration-centrifugation (centrifugal filters Amicon Ultra-4 with 100 kDa molecular weight cut-off, Millipore, Germany). Briefly, 500 µL of each HCT-loaded nanoparticle dispersion was put into the upper chamber of the ultrafiltration device, and then centrifuged at 12,000 rpm for 30 min. The concentration of unincorporated drug in the aqueous phase, collected in the outer chamber of the ultrafiltration device, was then spectrometrically assayed at 272 nm (UV–vis 1600 Shimadzu spectrophotometer, Tokyo, Japan). Entrapment efficiency (EE%) of HCT in nanoparticles was calculated according to the following equation:

$$EE\% = \frac{W_{total\ drug} - W_{free\ drug}}{W_{total\ drug}} \times 100$$

where $W_{free\ drug}$ is the amount of unincorporated drug in the aqueous phase after ultrafiltration-centrifugation. Any interference from other components was observed.

2.5. In Vitro Drug Release

In vitro drug release experiments from SLN and NLC were conducted according to the dialysis bag technique [22]. Dialysis bags of cellulose acetate (12,500 cut-off, Sigma-Aldrich, St. Louis, MO, USA) were soaked 12 h in pH 4.5 gastric buffer and then filled with 1 mL of SLN or NLC dispersion. The bags were then immersed, 2 h in 100 mL of pH 4.5 phosphate buffer mimicking the infant gastric pH (HCT solubility in the medium 0.7 mg/mL) and after 3 h in 100 mL of pH 6.8 phosphate buffer (mimicking the intestinal pH), both at 37 °C, under magnetic stirring at 50 rpm. The amount of released drug in the acceptor compartment was UV assayed at 272 nm at given time intervals. Each withdrawn sample was replaced with an equal volume of fresh medium, and a correction for the cumulative dilution was made. Experiments were carried out in triplicate.

Drug release data were fitted into different kinetic models (zero-order, first-order, Higuchi and Korsmeyer–Peppas), in order to find the best fitting kinetic model. The prevalent mechanism of drug release from SLN and NLC samples was also inferred from the value of the diffusional release exponent (n) of the Korsmeyer–Peppas equation:

$$F_t = k \times t^n$$

where F_t is the drug fraction released at time t, k the release constant, n the diffusional exponent.

The values of n indicate the mechanism of drug release: $n < 0.5$: Fickian diffusion; $0.5 < n < 0.9$: non-Fickian transport (anomalous transport), and $n > 0.9$: type-II transport.

2.6. Storage Stability Studies of Selected Lipid Nanoparticles

All the selected drug-loaded SLN and NLC dispersions were stored at 4 ± 1 °C for 6 months and checked every 30 days for mean particle size, PDI and zeta potential (Zetasizer Nano ZS, Malvern Instruments Ltd., Malvern, UK). At the end of the storage period, samples were also checked for drug EE%, to evaluate the entity of drug expulsion phenomena. At least three replicate analyses were done for each sample. Possible crystallization, precipitation, mold formation or gelling phenomena were also checked by visual inspection.

2.7. Cytotoxicity and Cellular Uptake Studies

Caco-2, a human colorectal adenocarcinoma cell line obtained from American Type Culture Collection (ATCC, Rockville, MD, USA), was cultured in Dulbecco's Modified Eagle's medium (DMEM, Euroclone, Milan, Italy), supplemented with 20% fetal bovine serum (FBS), 1% L-glutamine and 1% Penicillin/Streptomycin (all Carlo Erba reagents, Milan, Italy) at 37 °C in an atmosphere containing 5% CO_2. HCT was dissolved in dimethylsulfoxide (DMSO) and, then, diluted in DMEM in order to obtain the appropriate concentrations to be tested. The final concentration of DMSO was <0.1%.

For viability test, Caco-2 cells were seeded in 96-well plates at a density of 5×10^3 cells/well in 100 µL of medium. After 24 h of incubation at 37 °C in 5% CO_2, the cells were exposed to the formulations, with or without HCT (1:50, 1:100 or 1:200), for 24 h. Cell viability was assessed by a colorimetric method based on reduction of 3-(4,5-dimethylthiazol-2-yl)-5-(3-carboxymethoxyphenyl)-2-(4-sulfophenyl)-2H-tetrazolium, inner salt (MTS, Promega Corporation, Madison, WI, USA). The optical density of the colored formazan product formed by MTS reduction was measured at 490 nm using a VICTOR^3 Wallac 1421 Multilabel Plate Reader (Perkin Elmer, Ramsey, NJ, USA). Data were expressed as a percentage of viable cells compared to cells exposed to the solvent alone.

For cellular uptake studies, SLN or NLC dispersions were labeled with rhodamine as fluorescence marker, by adding it to the lipid phase to obtain a final concentration of 10^{-5} M. Caco-2 cells were growth on glass cover-slips placed into 4-well plates for 24 h, then the labeled SLN and NLC were added, after 1:50 dilution, and maintained for 1 h at room temperature. After incubation time, cells were washed four times with pH 7.4 phosphate buffer solution (PBS) and fixed in 4% formaldehyde in 0.1 mol/L PBS for 10 min at room temperature. After fixation, cells were washed four times with PBS and cell nuclei were stained with 40,6-diamidino-2-phenylindole (DAPI) for 10 min at room temperature. The cells were washed once with PBS and the glass cover-slips were glued to glass microscope slides and observed by the Olympus BX63 microscope equipped with a Metal Halide Lamp (Prior Scientific Instruments Ltd., Cambridge, United Kingdom) and a digital camera Olympus XM 10 (Olympus, Milan, Italy). Ten photomicrographs were randomly taken for each sample and fluorescence was measured using ImageJ 1.33 image analysis software (freely available at http://rsb.info.nih.gov/ij, accessed on 23 March 2021).

2.8. Statistical Analysis

Statistical analysis of data was carried out according to the one-way analysis of variance. Differences between groups were tested by one-way ANOVA with Student-Newman-Keuls comparison post hoc test (GraphPad Prism version 6.0 Software, San Diego, CA, USA). Data were expressed as mean ± SD. A p value < 0.05 was considered significant.

3. Results and Discussion

3.1. Screening of Solid and Liquid Lipids for SLN and NLC Development

A preliminary screening for a proper selection of the solid and liquid lipids to be used for HCT-loaded SLNs and NLCs development was initially performed. It was based on the assessment of the solubility of HCT in the different examined solid and liquid lipids, since this is considered a critical condition for obtaining a good drug loading in the final nanoparticles. The results, in terms of transparency or turbidity of the different solutions after addition of 100 mg of drug to 5 g of melted lipid or 5 mL of liquid lipid, are collected in Table 1. When a transparent solution was obtained, a further 100 mg of drug was added, to achieve the target concentration of 0.2% w/v in the final formulation. Among solid lipids, Geleol® and Imwitor® 491 showed a certain solubilizing power towards HCT but only

Precirol® ATO5 allowed the total dissolution of this HCT amount, and, among liquid lipids, transparent solutions were obtained only with Transcutol® HP and Transcutol® P.

Table 1. HCT solubility in melted solid lipids (65 °C), and in liquid lipids heated at 65 °C in terms of solution transparency or turbidity (100 or 200 mg drug added to 5 g of melted solid lipid or 5 mL of liquid lipid).

Solid Lipid	Appearance of the Solution after Addition of		Liquid Lipid	Appearance of the Solution after Addition of	
	100 mg HCT	200 mg HCT		100 mg HCT	200 mg HCT
Precirol® ATO5	transparent	transparent	Labrafac® WL1349	turbid	
Compritol® 888ATO	turbid		Labrasol®	transparent	turbid
Geleol®	transparent	turbid	Labrasol® ALF	transparent	turbid
Cetyl Palmitate	turbid		Transcutol® HP	transparent	transparent
Tripalmitin	turbid		Transcutol® P	transparent	transparent
Imwitor® 491	transparent	turbid	Miglyol® 810N	turbid	
			Miglyol® 812	turbid	

Based on the results of solubility studies, Precirol® ATO5 was confirmed as the best solid lipid solubilizer for HCT [22] and was then selected for preparation of both SLN and NLC formulations.

On the other hand, Transcutol® HP was selected as the liquid lipid for NLC preparation, due to its higher solvent properties towards the drug than the other tested substances, and it was preferred to Transcutol® P due to its higher purity. In fact, a review about the safety of Transcutol as pharmaceutical excipient proved that the toxicity previously related to high levels of this solvent in nonclinical studies carried out before 1990, is likely to be attributed to the presence of significant amounts of impurities, particularly ethylene glycol; on the contrary, subsequent, extensive literature data showed its long safe use as a vehicle and solvent by multiple routes [29].

Regarding the surfactants, Gelucire® 44/14, considering its amphiphilic nature (HLB 14), was tested as non-ionic surfactant both in alternative to Tween® 80 (HLB 15) and Pluronic® F68 (HLB < 24), used in previous studies [22,25,30–32], and also in combination with each of them at different ratios. Gelucire are versatile polymers, consisting in mixtures of glycerides with PEG esters of fatty acids, widely used in drug delivery with different applications, mainly depending on their HLB values [33]. Among the hydrophilic grades of this polymer, Gelucire® 44/14 has been successfully used to improve solubility and dissolution rate of several poorly soluble drugs [34–37], and it also showed safe absorption enhancer properties [38]. Gelucire® 44/14 is also present in different currently marketed oral lipid-based formulations and is included in the FDA list of inactive ingredients.

Compatibility studies performed by DSC on pure drug and the selected components of SLN and NLC formulations, both separately and in the different combinations used, allowed to rule out possible solid-state interactions and/or incompatibility problems between them, thus confirming their suitability for use (data not shown).

3.2. Preparation of Nanoparticles

Preliminary experiments showed that 5 min of high-shear homogenization was enough to obtain particles of nanometric dimensions, while an increase at 10 min of homogenization time did not give rise to a significant reduction in nanoparticle size. Then, 5 min was selected as homogenization time for all nanoparticle formulations.

A series of empty SLN and NLC formulations was then prepared, in order to investigate the effect of different formulation variables on the nanoparticle properties in terms of mean dimensions, homogeneity and Zeta potential.

In particular, in the case of SLN formulations, the effect of replacing 1.5% w/w of Tween® 80 or Pluronic® F68 with different amounts of Gelucire® 44/14 (from 1.5 up to 7% w/w), or of their combined use, as well as the effect, by keeping the Gelucire® 44/14 content constant at 3.5% w/w, of varying the Precirol® ATO5 amount (from 5 up to 20% w/w), were evaluated.

On the other hand, in the case of NLC formulations, the effect of variations of the liquid lipid Transcutol® HP content (from 0.5 up to 5% w/w) and of the use of Gelucire® 44/14 as non ionic surfactant instead of, or in combination with Tween® 80 or Pluronic® F68, was investigated.

The composition of the various SLN and NLC formulations is given in Tables 2 and 3.

Table 2. Composition (% w/w) of the different SLN colloidal dispersions in water.

Code	Solid Lipid Precirol ATO5	Surfactant Type		
		Pluronic F68	Tween 80	Gelucire
SLN_1	5	1.5	-	-
SLN_2	5	-	1.5	-
SLN_3	5	-	-	1.5
SLN_4	5	-	-	3.5
SLN_5	5	-	-	7.0
SLN_6	5	1.5	-	5
SLN_7	5	-	1.5	5
SLN_8	5	1.5	-	6
SLN_9	5	-	1.5	6
SLN_{10}	7.5	-	-	3.5
SLN_{11}	10	-	-	3.5
SLN_{12}	15	-	-	3.5
SLN_{13}	20	-	-	3.5

Table 3. Composition (% w/w) of the different NLC colloidal dispersions in water.

Code	Solid Lipid Precirol ATO5	Liquid Lipid Transcutol HP	Surfactant Type		
			Pluronic F68	Tween 80	Gelucire
NLC_1	5	0.5	1.5	-	-
NLC_2	5	1	1.5	-	-
NLC_3	5	3	1.5	-	-
NLC_4	5	5	1.5	-	-
NLC_5	5	0.5	-	1.5	-
NLC_6	5	1	-	1.5	-
NLC_7	5	3	-	1.5	-
NLC_8	5	5	-	1.5	-
NLC_9	5	0.5	-	-	3.5
NLC_{10}	5	1	-	-	3.5
NLC_{11}	5	3	-	-	3.5
NLC_{12}	5	5	-	-	3.5
NLC_{13}	5	0.5	1.5	-	3.5
NLC_{14}	5	0.5	-	1.5	3.5

3.3. Characterization of Nanoparticles Formulations

Particle size, polydispersity index (PDI) and Zeta potential (ZP) were selected as the parameters for nanoparticles characterization, since they represent important characteristics having a strong influence on the stability, release rate and biological performance of the nanoparticulate systems.

In particular, particle size is considered a marker of the system stability and it should maintain a narrow range during storage because an increase in particle size during storage periods indicates agglomeration and hence physical instability [39]. Moreover, it seems that small particle size (particularly below 300 nm) of the formulation should improve the drug bioavailability, providing a rapid action and leading to a significant increase in cellular uptake rate [40]. Among the main factors able to affect nanoparticles particle size, by keeping the preparation conditions constant, formulation composition, i.e., type of lipids and surfactants used, may play an important role [41].

PDI is another important index of the physical stability of nanosuspensions, representing the width of particle size distribution. Low PDI values (<0.3) indicate a narrow size distribution, whereas PDI values greater than 0.5 are index of poorly homogeneous systems [42].

Finally, Zeta potential, i.e., the nanoparticles surface charge, is closely related to stability of the nanoparticles suspension, hindering aggregation phenomena [43,44]. In general, ZP values around ±30 mV are suggested for assuring good stability under storage of nanoparticles only electrostatically stabilized. However, ZP values around ±20 mV are considered to be enough for nanoparticles whose stability is the resultant of a combination of electrostatic and steric stabilization [45].

3.3.1. Effect of Type and % of Surfactant on SLN Physicochemical Properties

As shown in Figure 1A, the mean diameter of SLNs obtained using Pluronic® F68 (SLN_1) was around 350 nm, significantly smaller than those with Tween® 80 (SLN_2) (above 550 nm). This finding, observed also by other authors [22,30,46], has been attributed to a different incorporation way of the two surfactant molecules in the external shell of the nanoparticles [47].

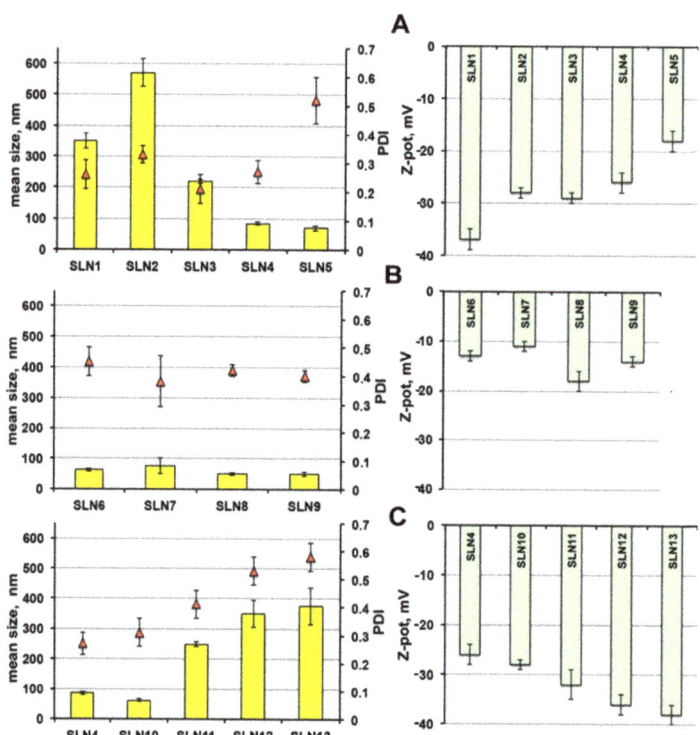

Figure 1. Physicochemical properties of empty SLNs in terms of mean size, polydispersity index (PDI) and Zeta potential: Scheme 1. SLN5 (**A**); SLN6-SLN9 (**B**); SLN10-SLN13 compared to SLN4 (**C**). See Table 2 for their composition.

The replacement of such surfactants with an equal amount (1.5%) of Gelucire® 44/14 (SLN_3), gave rise to very homogeneous nanoparticles of smaller dimensions, around 220 nm. A rise up to 3.5% of Gelucire® 44/14 content (SLN_4) resulted in a further clear particle size decrease, up to around 85 nm, probably due to the higher surfactant/lipid ratio [48]; good PDI and satisfactory ZP values were maintained. A further reduction of the nanoparticles dimensions (around 70 nm) was observed by increasing Gelucire® 44/14 content up to 7% (SLN_5), but it was accompanied by a PDI increase and a ZP decrease. Therefore, only SLN_4 formulation was selected for drug loading, together with SLN_1 and SLN_2 for comparison purpose.

The combined use of Gelucire® 44/14 with Pluronic® F68 or Tween® 80 (SLN_6-SLN_9), resulted in all cases in nanoparticles of very reduced dimensions, ranging from 75 to 50 nm (Figure 1B). However, while an acceptable homogeneity was maintained, a sensible reduction of ZP was observed, index of potential physical instability of the colloidal dispersion. For this reason, this formulation series was discarded and not considered for further studies.

Finally, the series of SLN formulations containing a fixed 3.5% Gelucire® 44/14 content and increasing amounts of the solid lipid Precirol® ATO5 (Figure 1C) showed that, after an initial particle size reduction for SLN containing 7.5% of solid lipid (SLN_{10}), a progressive increment of nanoparticles dimensions was instead observed when further rising its content, along with a PDI increase. This finding could be attributed to the concomitant decrease in the surfactant-to-lipid ratio [48]. Then, despite the favourable increment of the negative ZP value observed when increasing the Precirol® ATO5 content, formulations SLN_{11}, SLN_{12} and SLN_{13} were discarded and only SLN_{10} was selected for drug loading.

3.3.2. Effect of Surfactant Type and Liquid Lipid Amount on NLC Physical-Chemical Properties

As shown in Figure 2A, even in the case of NLCs, the use as surfactant of Tween® 80 (NLC_5-NLC_8) instead of Pluronic® F68 (NLC_1-NLC_4), gave rise to nanoparticles of greater mean size (around 500 vs. 350 nm), in agreement with previous results [25]. Moreover, for each NLC series, no significant variations of their dimensions, homogeneity and ZP were found with increasing the liquid lipid amount up to 5%.

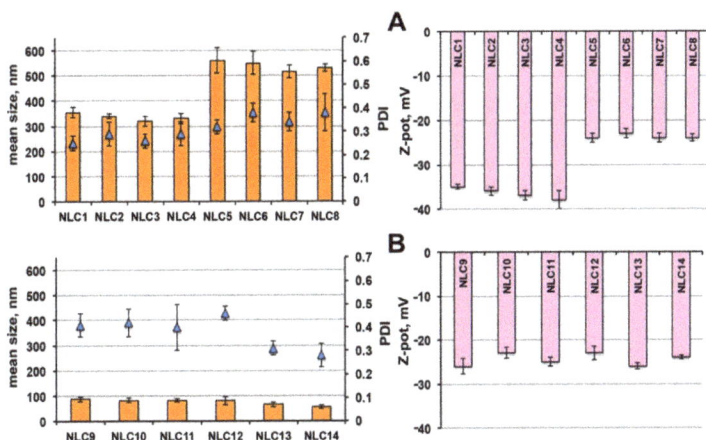

Figure 2. Physicochemical properties of empty NLCs in terms of mean size, polydispersity index (PDI) and Zeta potential: NLC_1-NLC_8 (**A**); NLC_9-NLC_{14} (**B**). See Table 3 for their composition.

Interestingly, the use of 3.5% Gelucire® 44/14 as surfactant (NLC_9-NLC_{12}) in place of Tween® 80 or Pluronic® F68 (Figure 2B), resulted in a marked reduction of nanoparticle dimensions (in all cases below 100 nm), with only a slight PDI increase. On the other hand, no advantages were observed in terms of nanoparticle size reduction or homogeneity improvement or ZP increase by enhancing the Transcutol® HP content from 0.5% (NLC_9) up to 5% (NLC_{12}).

A further decrease in nanoparticles size, accompanied by an improvement in homogeneity, was instead found when using Gelucire® 44/14 in combination with Pluronic®

F68 (NLC$_{13}$) or Tween80 (NLC$_{14}$), by keeping the liquid lipid amount constant at 0.5%. On the contrary, the kind of surfactant did not affect the ZP, which always ranged between −23 and −26 mV. These values can be considered sufficient to assure a good stability of the colloidal dispersions, in virtue of the presence of the steric-stabilizing surfactants [47].

Therefore, based on these results, and in order to minimize the use of Transcutol® HP, formulations NLC$_1$, NLC$_5$ and NLC$_9$ were selected for drug loading, containing, respectively, Pluronic® F68, Tween® 80 and Gelucire® 44/14 as surfactant and all containing the lowest liquid lipid content (0.5%). Formulations NLC$_{13}$ and NLC$_{14}$, containing Gelucire® 44/14 in mixture with Pluronic® F68 and Tween® 80, respectively, were also selected, due to their favourable properties in terms of very small particle size (around 60 nm), together with high homogeneity (PDI < 0.3) of the colloidal dispersion.

3.3.3. Characterization of Drug-Loaded SLNs and NLCs

The effect of drug loading on the physicochemical properties of the selected SLN and NLC formulations is presented in Figure 3A,B, where the letter L was added to the code of loaded formulations, to distinguish them from the corresponding empty ones. As expected, drug loading gave rise to a particle size increase, which was, however, limited, never exceeding 10% with respect to the corresponding empty nanoparticles. Moreover, no important variations were observed regarding the colloidal dispersion homogeneity, in terms of PDI values, or of the vesicle stability, in terms of surface charge, suggesting in all cases the obtainment of physically stable colloidal dispersion, substantially unaffected by drug loading.

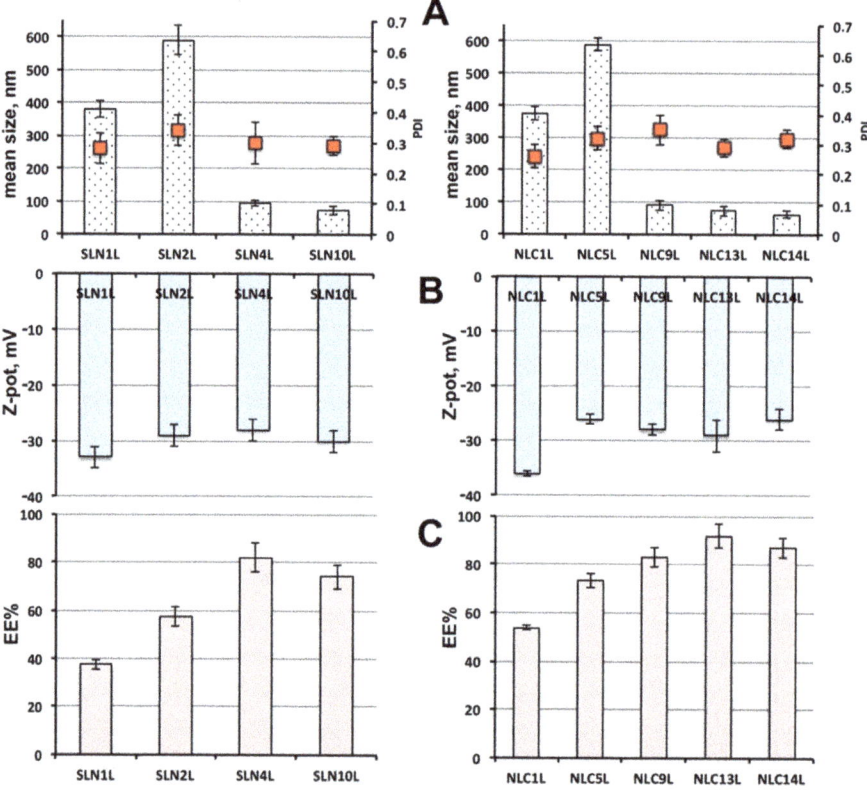

Figure 3. Physicochemical properties of the selected HCT-loaded SLN (left side, SLNnL) and NLC (right side, NLCnL) formulations: mean size and polydispersity index (PDI) (**A**), Zeta potential (**B**) and entrapment efficiency (EE%) (**C**).

As for the entrapment efficiency of SLN formulations (Figure 3C), the use as non-ionic surfactant of 3.5% Gelucire® 44/14 (SLN_4L), rather than 1.5% Pluronic® F68 (SLN_1L) or Tween® 80 (SLN_2L), resulted in an increase in EE% of 2.1 and 1.4 times, respectively, reaching about 80%. A smaller increase (1.8 and 1.2 times, respectively) was instead observed for $SLN_{10}L$ formulation, containing the same amount of Gelucire® 44/14, but a higher content of the solid lipid Precirol® ATO5 (7.5 vs. 5%), which probably negatively affected the drug incorporation ability of the nanoparticles.

Even in the case of NLC formulations, the replacement of Pluronic® F68 (NLC_1L) or Tween® 80 (NLC_5L) with 3.5% Gelucire® 44/14 (NLC_9L) enabled an entrapment efficiency improvement, by about 1.5 and 1.1 fold, respectively, overcoming 80%. A further EE% enhancement was obtained for NLC formulations containing Gelucire® 44/14 in mixture with Pluronic® F68 ($NLC_{13}L$) or Tween® 80 ($NLC_{14}L$), which, respectively, approached and even exceeded 90%.

Finally, by comparing the results obtained with the different SLNs and NLCs formulations, rather similar findings were observed in terms of size, PDI and Zeta potential of the nanoparticles. On the contrary, the better performance of NLCs in terms of entrapment efficiency appeared evident, due to the less ordered structure of this kind of lipid nanoparticles, compared to SLNs, which enabled them to incorporate greater drug amounts.

3.4. Release Studies

The HCT release curves from the selected SLN and NLC formulations are shown in Figure 4, together with that from the simple drug suspension, for comparison purposes.

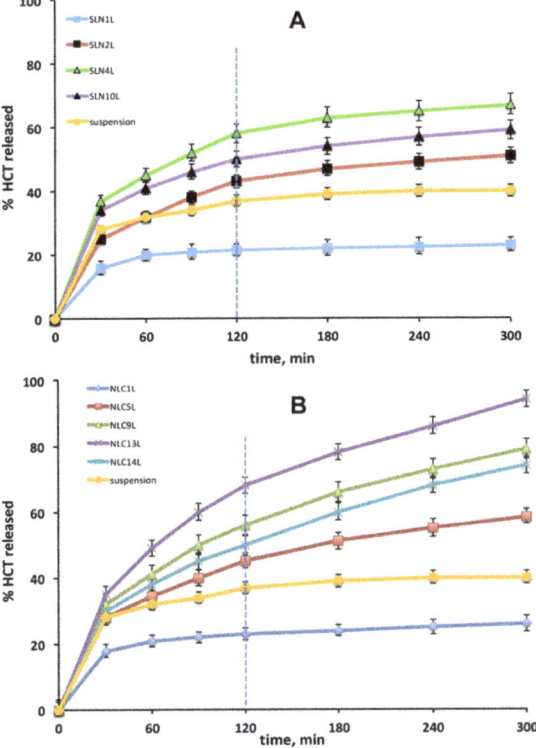

Figure 4. HCT release curves from the selected SLNnL (**A**) and NLCnL (**B**) formulations, at 37 °C for 2 h in pH 4.5 and 3 h in pH 6.8, together with that of the simple HCT suspension as reference.

The HCT suspension exhibited an initial fast release phase, due to the diffusion of the fraction of already dissolved drug; however, it was rapidly followed by a slow release phase, due to the very low drug solubility, reaching about 40% drug released at the end of the test.

Regarding NLCs formulations (Figure 4B), similarly to what observed for SLNs formulations, NLCs containing Pluronic® F68 (NLC_1L) exhibited a reduced release rate compared to the drug suspension, while an opposite result was given by Tween® 80-based NLC formulation (NLC_5L), which reached about 60% drug released at 5 h. This behaviour was analogous to that previously reported for analogous NLCs formulations, containing castor oil instead of Transcutol® HP as liquid lipid [25], and once again supported the critical role played by the surfactant type in affecting the drug release profile from lipid nanoparticles.

As found for SLNs formulations, the use of Gelucire® 44/14 as surfactant (NLC_9L) resulted in a clear improvement of the drug release rate, achieving nearly 80% of drug released at 5 h. Interestingly, a further release rate increase was given by NLC formulations containing Gelucire® 44/14 in mixture with Tween® 80 ($NLC_{13}L$), which showed a total drug amount released at the end of the test of about 95%. On the contrary, a slight decrease in drug delivery rate was observed when Pluronic® F68 was added in mixture to Gelucire® 44/14 ($NLC_{14}L$).

Finally, by comparing the global results obtained with the two series of lipid nanoparticles formulations, it appears evident that more regular and faster release profiles were generally provided by NLC than from SLN formulations. In particular, the best NLC formulations allowed a drug release rate 1.4 times higher than the best SLN formulation. This effect may be ascribed to the different physical state of the lipids in the two kinds of nanoparticles. In fact, in the case of SLNs, the lipids are more densely and ordinately packed, thus hindering the drug release, while the less ordered and less crystalline structure of NLC can facilitate and improve drug delivery [49].

Kinetic evaluation of drug release profiles from the different SLNs and NLCs was also performed, in order to obtain some insight about the prevalent mechanisms governing drug release from the delivery system. Release data were fitted into the most common release kinetic models: zero order, first order, Higuchi and Korsmeyer–Peppas models. The obtained values of correlation coefficients (R^2) and release exponent (n), summarized in Table 4, indicated that SLNs followed Korsmeyer–Peppas release kinetic, while NLCs release data well fitted with both Higuchi and Korsmeyer–Peppas kinetic models. In any case, n values <0.5 were obtained in all cases, indicating a predominantly diffusion-controlled mechanism of drug release. Moreover, the initial burst release observed during the first 30 min can be due to the diffusion of drug present on the nanoparticle outer surface, and might provide a fast onset of action.

Table 4. Correlation coefficients (R^2) and release exponent (n) values obtained from the different kinetic models for SLNs (upper) and NLCs (down) formulations.

Kinetic Model	SLN_1L	SLN_2L	SLN_4L	$SLN_{10}L$	
Zero order	0.9239	0.8713	0.8578	0.9236	
First order	0.927	0.8989	0.8995	0.9483	
Higuchi	0.964	0.9313	0.9214	0.9690	
Kormeyer-Peppas	0.9842	0.9538	0.9509	0.9862	
Kormeyer-Peppas (n)	0.08	0.28	0.24	0.22	
Kinetic model	NLC_1L	NLC_5L	NLC_9L	$NLC_{13}L$	$NLC_{14}L$
Zero order	0.9771	0.9527	0.9675	0.9639	0.9853
First order	0.9797	0.9756	0.9881	0.9751	0.9897
Higuchi	0.9955	0.9866	0.9940	0.9913	0.9992
Kormeyer-Peppas	0.9958	0.9939	0.9963	0.9933	0.9994
Kormeyer-Peppas (n)	0.13	0.33	0.40	0.39	0.42

Considering all of the obtained results, in terms of physico-chemical properties, entrapment efficiency and drug release behaviour, SLN$_4$L, NLC$_9$L, NLC$_{13}$L, and NLC$_{14}$L were ultimately selected as the best formulations of the two series of colloidal dispersions and subjected to further studies to evaluate their stability under storage and their actual safety.

3.5. Storage Stability Studies

The physical stability of the selected SLN and NLC formulations was monitored during 6 months of storage at 4 °C. The simple visual inspection did not evidence any phenomenon of drug precipitation, or crystallization process or formation of mold.

The physicochemical properties of the colloidal dispersions were evaluated in terms of variations in mean dimensions, homogeneity (PDI) and surface charge of the nanoparticles (Figure 5). In all cases, no significant changes in the values of such parameters ($p > 0.05$) were detected during the whole storage period with respect to the freshly prepared systems. Thus, these results were considered indicative of the good physical stability of all the colloidal dispersion systems considered.

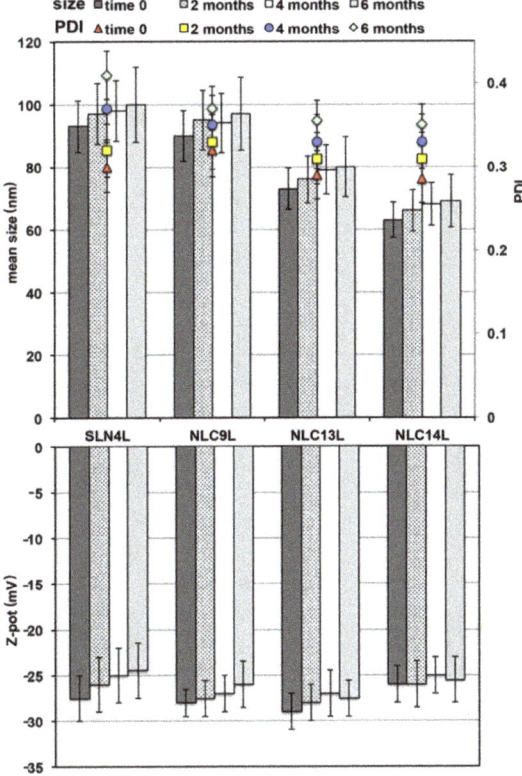

Figure 5. Effect of storage at 4 ± 1 °C on mean size, PDI and Zeta potential of the selected SLN and NLC formulations.

At the end of the storage period, a check of the EE% of the selected formulations was also performed. In the case of all NLC formulations, only a slight, not significant ($p > 0.05$) reduction was observed, that never exceeded 5%. On the contrary, a more evident and significant ($p < 0.05$) decrease in the amount of encapsulated drug was found for SLN$_4$L formulation, which reached an about 15% of drug leakage after 6 months storage at 4 °C. These results confirmed the lower tendency to drug expulsion phenomena during the storage of NLCs with respect to SLNs, in virtue of their less ordered nature, due to the presence of the liquid lipid within the solid lipid structure [24].

3.6. Cytotoxicity and Cellular Uptake Studies

The cytotoxicity of the developed SLN and NLC formulations was assessed by MTS cell assay. Cell viability was determined after 24 h exposure of Caco-2 cells to empty or HCT-loaded SLN and NLC formulations or to a solution of plain drug, all at three different dilutions. The results of this study, reported in Figure 6 as a percentage of cell viability compared to that of control cells exposed to the solvent alone, proved that none of the evaluated SLN and NLC formulations, both empty or drug-loaded, exhibited a cytotoxicity, at all dilutions tested. In fact, in all cases, a cell viability close to 100% was maintained, similar to that of the control (pure solvent) or of the HCT simple solution. A slight reduction of up to approximately 95% was observed only for the drug-loaded NLC_9 and NLC_{13} formulations, only at the lowest dilution (1:50) but this effect was not statistically significant compared to the control ($p > 0.05$). These results further highlighted the importance of a proper surfactants selection. Biocompatible surfactants are in fact highly preferable to minimize any potential surfactant-induced toxicity of lipid nanocarriers [50].

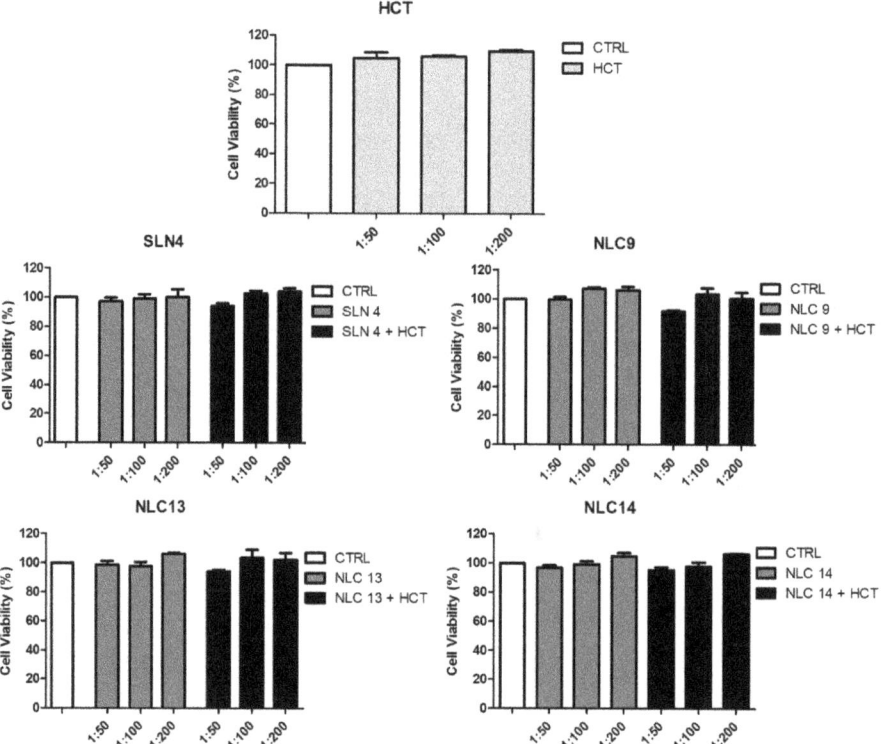

Figure 6. Cytotoxicity on CaCo-2 cell line expressed as cell viability % of pure HCT, empty and drug-loaded SLN4, empty and drug-loaded NLC9, NLC13, NLC14 at different dilutions (1:50, 1:100, 1:200) after 24 h exposure.

Cellular uptake experiments were performed to test the actual internalization of SLN and NLC formulations into intestinal epithelium. To this aim, Caco-2 cells were incubated with SLN and NLCs labeled with rhodamine as fluorescent dye. After 1 h of exposure, an evident intracellular staining was observed in all cases, demonstrating that all formulations were able to enter Caco-2 intestinal cells, even though some differences in intensity of the effect were observed among the different formulations, NLC13 and NLC14 being the most effective ones, probably due to their smaller size and/or the combination of two different surfactants (Figure 7).

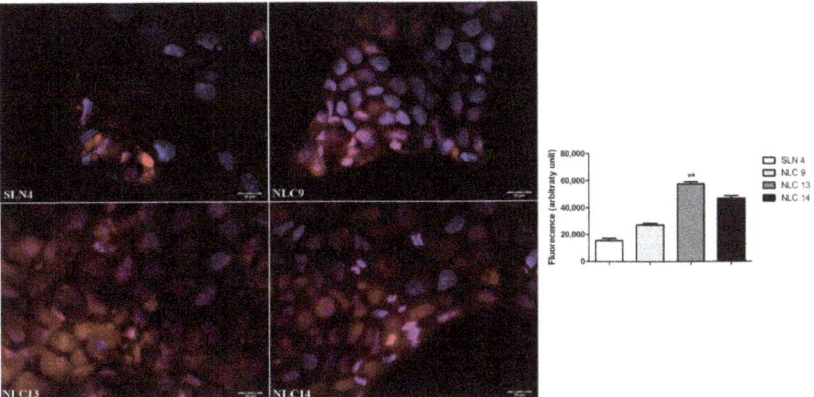

Figure 7. Cellular uptake of rhodamine-labeled SLN and NLC in Caco-2 cells after 1 h of exposure at 37 °C. Nuclei stained with DAPI. Final magnification 20×, scale bar 50 µm. Results expressed as mean ± SEM, $n = 10$; ** $p < 0.01$ vs. SLN4 (Kruskal–Wallis test and Dunn's multiple comparisons test).

4. Conclusions

Careful investigations about the choice of the most effective solid and liquid lipid components as well as surfactants for the development of new SLN and NLC-based HCT pediatric formulations were successful in further improving their performance with respect to previously developed formulations [22,25] in terms of particle size, entrapment efficiency, drug release properties and storage stability.

In fact, in the case of SLN formulations, the use of Gelucire® 44/14 (rather than Pluronic® F68 or Tween® 80) yielded a marked reduction of the particle size up to 95–75 nm (with respect to around 600–400 nm), and at the same time an improvement in entrapment efficiency, reaching about 80% (with respect to 40 or 60%, respectively) as well as in drug release rate, reaching about 65% of HCT released after 300 min (versus 20 or 50%, respectively). On the other hand, in case of NLC formulations, the use of Gelucire® 44/14, alone (NLC_9L), or in combination with Pluronic® F68 or Tween® 80 ($NLC_{13}L$ and $NLC_{14}L$, respectively), allowed also in this case a dramatic reduction of particle size up to 90, 75 and 65 nm, respectively (compared to around 400 or 600 nm of NLC_1L or NLC_5L containing PluronicF68 or Tween® 80 alone, respectively), maintaining a similar entrapment efficiency, around 90%, while improving drug release rate, reaching more than 90% of HCT released after 300 min (versus 25 or 60%).

A comparison between the selected SLN (SLN_4L and $SLN_{10}L$) and NLC (NLC_9L, $NLC_{13}L$ and $NLC_{14}L$) formulations confirmed the superior performance of the latter in terms of drug entrapment efficiency and drug release behaviour. Similar results were instead obtained in stability studies, where all the examined formulations maintained almost unchanged their properties in terms of particle size, PDI and zeta potential, without any apparent variations of organoleptic properties nor mold formation after 6 months storage at 4 °C. However, a more evident drug leakage phenomenon was found for SLN (15%) than for all NLCs (<5%)

Importantly, none of the new developed SLN and NLC HCT formulations showed signs of cytotoxicity on Caco-2 cells, used as model of human intestinal cells, confirming the safety of the employed excipients. Finally, cellular uptake studies proved that all the selected formulations were able to enter Caco-2 intestinal cells thus increasing HCT intestinal permeability.

Author Contributions: Conceptualization, C.L. and M.C.; Data curation, F.M., M.D., C.L. and M.C.; Formal analysis, M.D.; Investigation, F.M. and M.C.; Methodology, F.M. and M.D.; Project administration, P.M.; Supervision, P.M. and C.L.; Writing—original draft, P.M.; Writing—review & editing, P.M. and M.C. All authors have read and agreed to the published version of the manuscript.

Funding: This research received no external funding.

Institutional Review Board Statement: Not applicable.

Informed Consent Statement: Not applicable.

Data Availability Statement: Not applicable.

Conflicts of Interest: The authors declare no conflict of interest.

References

1. *Paediatric Addendum to the Note for Guidance on the Clinical Investigation on Medicinal Products in the Treatment of Hypertension—EMA/CHMP/206815/2013*; European Medicines Agency, Committee for Medicinal Products for Human Use (CHMP): Amsterdam, The Netherlands, 2015.
2. WHO Model List of Essential Medicines for Children, 4th List, April 2013. Available online: http://www.who.int/medicines/publications/essentialmedicines/en/index.html (accessed on 18 September 2018).
3. National High Blood Pressure Education Program Working Group on High Blood Pressure in Children and Adolescents. The Fourth Report on the Diagnosis, Evaluation, and Treatment of High Blood Pressure in Children and Adolescents. *Pediatrics* **2004**, *114*, 555–576. [CrossRef]
4. Claxton, A.J.; Cramer, J.; Pierce, C. A systematic review of the associations between dose regimens and medication compliance. *Clin. Ther.* **2001**, *23*, 1296–1310. [CrossRef]
5. Amidon, G.L.; Lennernäs, H.; Shah, V.P.; Crison, J.R. A Theoretical Basis for a Biopharmaceutic Drug Classification: The Correlation of in Vitro Drug Product Dissolution and in Vivo Bioavailability. *Pharm. Res.* **1995**, *12*, 413–420. [CrossRef] [PubMed]
6. Reddy, B.B.K.; Karunakar, A. Biopharmaceutics Classification System: A Regulatory Approach. *Dissolut. Technol.* **2011**, *18*, 31–37. [CrossRef]
7. Patel, R.B.; Patel, U.R.; Rogge, M.C.; Shah, V.P.; Prasad, V.K.; Selen, A.; Welling, P.G. Bioavailability of Hydrochlorothiazide from Tablets and Suspensions. *J. Pharm. Sci.* **1984**, *73*, 359–361. [CrossRef]
8. Mollica, J.A.; Rehm, C.R.; Smith, J.B. Hydrolysis of Hydrochlorothiazide. *J. Pharm. Sci.* **1969**, *58*, 635–636. [CrossRef]
9. Mollica, J.A.; Rehm, C.R.; Smith, J.B.; Govan, H.K. Hydrolysis of Benzothiadiazines. *J. Pharm. Sci.* **1971**, *60*, 1380–1384. [CrossRef]
10. Tagliari, M.P.; Stuzler, S.K.; Assreuy, J.; Bresolin, T.M.B.; Silva, M.A.S. Evaluation of physicochemical characteristics of suspensions containing hydrochlorotiazide developed for pediatric use. *Lat. Am. J. Pharm.* **2009**, *28*, 734–740.
11. Mahajan, A.A.; Thaker, A.K.; Mohanraj, K. LC, LC-MS/MS studies for the identification and characterization of degradation products of hydrochlorothiazide and establishment of mechanistic approach towards degradation. *J. Braz. Chem. Soc.* **2012**, *23*, 445–452. [CrossRef]
12. Batchelor, H.K.; Marriott, J.F. Formulations for children: Problems and solutions. *Br. J. Clin. Pharmacol.* **2015**, *79*, 405–418. [CrossRef]
13. Richey, R.H.; Shah, U.U.; Peak, M.; Craig, J.V.; Ford, J.L.; Barker, C.E.; Nunn, A.J.; Turner, M.A. Manipulation of drugs to achieve the required dose is intrinsic to paediatric practice but is not supported by guidelines or evidence. *BMC Pediatr.* **2013**, *13*. [CrossRef] [PubMed]
14. Zahn, J.; Hoerning, A.; Trollmann, R.; Rascher, W.; Neubert, A. Manipulation of Medicinal Products for Oral Administration to Paediatric Patients at a German University Hospital: An Observational Study. *Pharmaceutics* **2020**, *12*, 583. [CrossRef]
15. Fabiano, V.; Mameli, C.; Zuccotti, G.V. Paediatric pharmacology: Remember the excipients. *Pharm. Res.* **2011**, *63*, 362–365. [CrossRef] [PubMed]
16. Valeur, K.S.; Holst, H.; Allegaert, K. Excipients in Neonatal Medicinal Products: Never Prescribed, Commonly Administered. *Pharm. Med.* **2018**, *32*, 251–258. [CrossRef]
17. Chakraborty, S.; Shukla, D.; Mishra, B.; Singh, S. Lipid-an emerging platform for oral delivery of drugs with poor bioavailability. *Eur. J. Pharm. Biopharm.* **2009**, *73*, 1–15. [CrossRef] [PubMed]
18. Lim, S.B.; Banerjee, A.; Onyuksel, H. Improvement of drug safety by the use of lipid-based nanocarriers. *J. Control. Release* **2012**, *163*, 34–45. [CrossRef] [PubMed]
19. Mukherjee, S.; Ray, S.; Thakur, R.S. Solid lipid nanoparticles: A modern formulation approach in drug delivery system. *Indian J. Pharm. Sci.* **2009**, *71*, 349–358. [CrossRef]
20. Mehnert, W.; Mäder, K. Solid lipid nanoparticles. *Adv. Drug Deliv. Rev.* **2012**, *64*, 83–101. [CrossRef]
21. Silva, A.C.; Kumar, A.; Wild, W.; Ferreira, D.; Santos, D.; Forbes, B. Long-term stability, biocompatibility and oral delivery potential of risperidone-loaded solid lipid nanoparticles. *Int. J. Pharm.* **2012**, *436*, 798–805. [CrossRef]

22. Cirri, M.; Mennini, N.; Maestrelli, F.; Mura, P.; Ghelardini, C.; Di Cesare Mannelli, L. Development and in vivo evaluation of an innovative "Hydrochlorothiazide-in Cyclodextrins-in Solid Lipid Nanoparticles" formulation with sustained release and enhanced oral bioavailability for potential hypertension treatment in pediatrics. *Int. J. Pharm.* **2017**, *521*, 73–83. [CrossRef]
23. Müller, R.H.; Radtke, M.; Wissing, S.A. Nanostructured lipid matrices for improved microencapsulation of drugs. *Int. J. Pharm.* **2002**, *242*, 121–128. [CrossRef]
24. Beloqui, A.; Solinís, M.Á.; Rodríguez-Gascó, A.; Almeida, A.J.; Préat, V. Nanostructured lipid carriers: Promising drug delivery systems for future clinics. *Nanomed. Nanotechnol. Biol. Med.* **2016**, *12*, 143–161. [CrossRef] [PubMed]
25. Cirri, M.; Maestrini, L.; Maestrelli, F.; Mennini, N.; Mura, P.; Ghelardini, C.; Di Cesare Mannelli, L. Design, characterization and in vivo evaluation of Nanostructured Lipid Carriers (NLC) as a new drug delivery system for hydrochlorothiazide oral administration in pediatric therapy. *Drug Deliv.* **2018**, *25*, 1910–1921. [CrossRef]
26. Kasongo, K.W.; Pardeike, J.; Müller, R.H.; Walker, R.B. Selection and characterization of suitable lipid excipients for use in the manufacture of didanosine-loaded solid lipid nanoparticles and nanostructured lipid carriers. *J. Pharm. Sci.* **2011**, *100*, 5185–5196. [CrossRef]
27. Nnamani, P.O.; Hansen, S.; Windbergs, M.; Lehr, C.-M. Development of artemether-loaded nanostructured lipid carrier (NLC) formulation for topical application. *Int. J. Pharm.* **2014**, *477*, 208–217. [CrossRef]
28. Cirri, M.; Bragagni, M.; Mennini, N.; Mura, P. Development of a new delivery system consisting in "drug-in cyclodextrin-in nanostructured lipid carriers" for ketoprofen topical delivery. *Eur. J. Pharm. Biopharm.* **2012**, *80*, 46–53. [CrossRef] [PubMed]
29. Sullivan, D.W., Jr.; Gad, S.C.; Julien, M. A review of the nonclinical safety of Transcutol®, a highly purified form of diethylene glycol monoethyl ether (DEGEE) used as a pharmaceutical excipient. *Food Chem. Toxicol.* **2014**, *72*, 40–50. [CrossRef] [PubMed]
30. Cirri, M.; Maestrelli, F.; Mura, P.; Ghelardini, C.; Di Cesare Mannelli, L. Combined Approach of Cyclodextrin Complexation and Nanostructured Lipid Carriers for the Development of a Pediatric Liquid Oral Dosage Form of Hydrochlorothiazide. *Pharmaceutics* **2018**, *10*, 287. [CrossRef]
31. Gaspar, D.P.; Faria, V.; Goncalves, L.M.D.; Taboada, P.; Remunan-Lopez, C.; Almeida, A.J. Rifabutin-loaded solid lipid nanoparticles for inhaled antitubercular therapy: Physicochemical and in vitro studies. *Int. J. Pharm.* **2016**, *497*, 199–209. [CrossRef]
32. Padhye, S.G.; Nagarsenker, M.S. Simvastatin Solid Lipid Nanoparticles for Oral Delivery: Formulation Development and In vivo Evaluation. *Indian J. Pharm. Sci.* **2013**, *75*, 591–598.
33. Panigrahi, K.C.; Patra, C.N.; Jena, K.G.; Ghose, D.; Jena, J.; Panda, S.K.; Sahu, M. Gelucire: A versatile polymer for modified release drug delivery system. *Future J. Pharm. Sci.* **2018**, *4*, 102–108. [CrossRef]
34. Kawakami, K.; Miyoshi, K.; Ida, Y. Solubilization behavior of poorly soluble drugs with combined use of Gelucire 44/14 and cosolvent. *J. Pharm. Sci.* **2004**, *93*, 1471–1479. [CrossRef]
35. Aparna, K.; Meenakshi, B.; Monika, S. Improvement of dissolution rate and solubility of nifedipine by formulation of solid dispersions. *Pharm. Res.* **2010**, *4*, 38–45.
36. Borhade, V.; Pathak, S.; Sharma, S.; Patravale, V. Clotrimazole nanoemulsion for malaria chemotherapy. Part I: Preformulation studies, formulation design and physicochemical evaluation. *Int. J. Pharm.* **2012**, *431*, 138–148. [CrossRef] [PubMed]
37. Da Fonseca Antunes, A.; Geest, B.; Vervaet, C.; Remon, J.P. Gelucire 44/14 based immediate release formulations for poorly water-soluble drugs. *Drug Dev. Ind. Pharm.* **2013**, *39*, 791–798. [CrossRef] [PubMed]
38. Zhang, H.; Huang, X.; Mi, J.; Huo, Y.; Xing, J.; Gao, Y. Improvement of pulmonary absorption of poorly absorbable drugs using Gelucire 44/14 as an absorption enhancer. *J. Pharm. Pharmacol.* **2014**, *66*, 1410–1420. [CrossRef] [PubMed]
39. Khosa, A.; Reddi, S.; Saha, R.N. Nanostructured lipid carriers for site-specific drug delivery. *Biomed. Pharmacother.* **2018**, *103*, 598–613. [CrossRef]
40. Andrysek, T. Impact of physical properties of formulations on bioavailability of active substance: Current and novel drugs with cyclosporine. *Mol. Immunol.* **2003**, *39*, 1061–1065. [CrossRef]
41. Üner, M. Characterization and imaging of Solid Lipid Nanoparticles and Nanostructured Lipid Carriers. In *Handbook of Nanoparticles*; Aliofkhazraei, M., Ed.; Springer: Cham, Switzerland, 2016; pp. 117–141.
42. Lakshmi, P.; Kumar, G.A. Nanosuspension technology: A review. *Int. J. Pharm. Pharmaceut. Sci.* **2010**, *2*, 35–40.
43. Freitas, C.; Müller, R.H. Effect of light and temperature on zeta potential and physical stability in solid lipid nanoparticle (SLN^{TM}) dispersions. *Int. J. Pharm.* **1998**, *168*, 221–229. [CrossRef]
44. Müller, R.H.; Jacobs, C.; Kayser, O. Nanosuspensions as particulate drug formulations in therapy: Rationale for development and what we can expect for the future. *Adv. Drug Deliv. Rev.* **2001**, *47*, 3–19. [CrossRef]
45. Zimmermann, E.; Müller, R.H. Electrolyte- and pH-stabilities of aqueous solid lipid nanoparticle (SLN^{TM}) dispersions in artificial gastrointestinal media. *Eur. J. Pharm. Biopharm.* **2001**, *52*, 203–210. [CrossRef]
46. Bhupinder, K.; Newton, M.J. Impact of Pluronic® F68 vs Tween® 80 on fabrication and evaluation of acyclovir SLNs for skin delivery. *Recent Patents Drug Deliv. Formul.* **2016**, *10*, 1–15.
47. Radomska-Soukharev, A. Stability of lipid excipients in solid lipid nanoparticles. *Adv. Drug Del. Rev.* **2007**, *59*, 411–418. [CrossRef]
48. Gaba, B.; Fazil, M.; Ali, A.; Baboota, S.; Sahni, J.K.; Ali, J. Nanostructured lipid (NLCs) carriers as a bioavailability enhancement tool for oral administration. *Drug Deliv.* **2015**, *22*, 691–700. [CrossRef]

49. Aditya, N.P.; Macedo, A.S.; Doktorovová, S.; Souto, E.; Kim, S.; Chang, P.-S.; Ko, S. Development and evaluation of lipid nanocarriers for quercetin delivery: A comparative study of solid lipid nanoparticles (SLN), nanostructured lipid carriers (NLC), and lipid nanoemulsions (LNE). *LWT Food Sci. Technol.* **2014**, *59*, 115–121. [CrossRef]
50. Scioli Montoto, S.; Giuliana Muraca, G.; Ruiz, M.E. Solid Lipid Nanoparticles for Drug Delivery: Pharmacological and Biopharmaceutical Aspects. *Front. Mol. Biosci.* **2020**, *7*, 587997. [CrossRef] [PubMed]

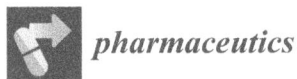 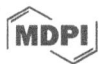

Article

Epidermal Delivery of Retinyl Palmitate Loaded Transfersomes: Penetration and Biodistribution Studies

Eloy Pena-Rodríguez, Mari Carmen Moreno, Bárbara Blanco-Fernandez, Jordi González and Francisco Fernández-Campos *

Topical & Oral development R+D Reig Jofre Laboratories, Gran Capitan Street 10, San Joan Despi, 08970 Barcelona, Spain; eloy.pena@reigjofre.com (E.P.-R.); maricarmen.moreno@reigjofre.com (M.C.M.); barbara.blanco.fernandez@gmail.com (B.B.-F.); jordi.gonzalez@reigjofre.com (J.G)
* Correspondence: Francisco.fernandez@reigjofre.com; Tel.: +34-935-507-718

Received: 16 December 2019; Accepted: 27 January 2020; Published: 30 January 2020

Abstract: The alteration of retinoids levels in the skin can cause different disorders in the maturation of epithelial skin cells. Topical administration of these lipophilic molecules is a challenge that can be addressed by encapsulation into drug delivery systems. In this study, retinyl palmitate transferosomes formulated in cream were developed and the increases in the penetration of the active ingredients as well as the biodistribution were evaluated in vitro and in vivo. Transfersomes demonstrated a significant increase in the administration of retinyl palmitate to the epidermis by quantification of the active ingredients in the different layers of the skin, as well as by fluorescence microscopy of biopsies of non-dermatomized pig-ear skin. These results suggest that transfersomes may be an efficient vehicle for the delivery of retinoids to inner layers of the skin, such as the epidermis.

Keywords: transfersomes; retinyl palmitate; biodistribution; skin; penetration; drug release

1. Introduction

Vitamin A derivatives are a group of lipid-soluble compounds including retinol, retinal, retinyl acetate, retinyl linoleate and retinyl palmitate (RP). Retinoids have important effects on skin cells. Retinoid levels in the skin are involved in the correct cellular maturation of keratinocytes, and when the skin is damaged, they induce keratinocyte proliferation and modulate epidermal differentiation [1]. Moreover, retinoids stimulate the production of extracellular matrix proteins such as collagen I by dermal fibroblasts. Alterations in these levels produce a de-structuring of corneocytes' layers and, consequently, an increase in transepidermal water loss. Retinoids can also lighten hyperpigmented skin by decreasing melanocyte tyrosinase activity, inhibit the sebocyte proliferation and lipid synthesis, and alter their keratin expression. Alterations in retinoids skin levels can cause skin dehydration, lack of elasticity, sebum overproduction and hyperpigmentation, among other effects [2,3].

As retinoids cannot be synthesized by the body, they must be supplied through other sources [4]. Since these molecules are easily degraded by oxidation or photodegradation, and they are very hydrophobic, their topical bioavailability when applied on the skin surface remains quite low. In addition, retinoids have adverse effects such as hepatotoxicity, changes in lipid metabolism and bone density, teratogenicity, and they can cause significant skin irritation. Most of these effects occur after oral administration. Regarding topical administration, the main adverse effects are phototoxicity and skin irritation. One plausible mechanism of phototoxicity may be related to the formation of free radicals after the exposure of retinoids to UV light that damages the DNA. Relevant clinical studies or studies in animal models are therefore needed to establish whether the pro-oxidant activity of photoexcited vitamin A is observed in vivo, and to assess the related risks [5].

Skin irritation is linked to retinoids due to its pharmacological effects through retinoic acid receptor signaling [6]. Cytokines such as IL-1, TNF-α, IL-6, and IL-8 are thought to be more important in retinoid-induced dermatitis [7]. Retinyl Palmitate was irritating to rabbits' skin, and a slight irritant to rabbit eyes. [4]. Thus, although retinoids have been classically incorporated into emulsions to overcome some of these limitations, skin irritation and photodegradability issues are still a problem [8]. The inclusion of retinol derivatives such as retinyl palmitate into nanocarriers for topical delivery is an interesting strategy that can lead to higher stability and enhance skin penetration [9]. Liposomes are a suitable choice for retinoids' encapsulation, as the active ingredients can be incorporated into the membrane of the particles, ending in skin penetration and enhanced stability.

Liposomes are spherical vesicles formed of a lipid bilayer and an aqueous cavity. They consist of phospholipids or synthetic amphiphilic molecules, usually combined with sterols to reduce their membrane permeability. Phospholipids tend to self-assemble in the presence of water due to their amphiphilic nature. The hydrophilic head is oriented towards the water, while the apolar tails are located in the inner part of the bilayer. The nature of the lipids will determine the liposomes' properties. Saturated phospholipids can obtain liposomes with a lower permeability and greater stability than unsaturated phospholipids [10].

Classic liposomes usually accumulate in the stratum corneum and skin annexes. Therefore, they are not a good means to reach deeper layers of the skin or for transdermal absorption [11]. Therefore, different liposomal approaches have appeared. One example of these are ethosomes, which have ethanol in the vesicle cavity that behaves as a penetration promoter [12]. Another example are transfersomes, which are ultra-deformable liposomes [13]. This type of liposome has an "edge activator" (i.e., sodium cholate, sodium deoxycholate, span 80, Tween 80 or dipotassium glycyrrhizinate, among others) in its lipid membrane that allows it to increase its elasticity. There are several theories that explain the high penetration ability of these vesicles. The most accepted theory is that the high deformability of the transfersomes allows them to cross the intercellular channels of the stratum corneum [14,15]. Several researchers have demonstrated the improvement in topical penetration, for example, with retinol in dermatomized human skin and the keratinocites 3D model [9], and with lidocaine-loaded transfersomes, in order to avoid a painful local anesthetic injection [16].

The bilayer lipid matrix of cell membranes is composed of a mixture of different lipids. Among them, there is a growing interest in sphingolipids due their effects on skin cellular processes. Ceramides are a structurally heterogeneous and complex group of sphingolipids. It is well known that ceramides play an essential role in structuring and maintaining the water permeability barrier function of the skin. Ceramides maintain the dense crystalline structure of the lamellar lipids that are arranged between the corneocytes. They represent the 50% of lipids in the stratum corneum [17]. The rest of the lipids of the stratum corneum are cholesterol and free fatty acids. Together, they keep the lamellar structure of the stratum corneum and the barrier function of healthy skin in good condition. However, most skin disorders that have a diminished barrier function present a decrease in total ceramide content, with some differences in the ceramide pattern. Alterations in ceramide III levels are related to different skin diseases. In psoriatic skin, ceramides III and VII show a significant decrease versus normal stratum corneum [18]. In patients with atopic dermatitis, a decrease in the amount of ceramide III has been demonstrated to be correlated with an increase in transepidermal water loss [19]. Formulations containing lipids identical to those in skin and, in particular, ceramide supplementation, could improve disturbed skin conditions. Several authors have introduced ceramides in lipid-based vesicles to deliver them into the skin to restore lipid composition and to improve altered skin permeability [20,21]. Exogenously supplied, short-chain ceramides, such as ceramide III, induced keratinocyte differentiation in vitro and reinforced the pro-differentiation effects of other drugs [17].

Based on the effects of ceramide III and retinyl palmitate, as previously described, the formulations in this study were designed to improve and maintain the skin's barrier properties. The aims of this work were the development and characterization of a ceramide III-based transfersome cream formulation encapsulating retinyl palmitate, and the study of RP biodistribution through the different skin layers.

2. Materials and Methods

2.1. Materials

Ceramide III (Evonik Nutrition & Care, Essen, Germany), α-Tocopherol (Merck Chemicals and life, Barcelona, Spain), phosphatidylcholine (Lipoid, Ludwigshafen, Germany), Tween 80 (Croda Iberica S.A., Barcelona, Spain), Retynil Palmitate and Ethanol Absolute (Scharlab S.L. Barcelona, Spain) and purified water (Inhouse) were used to formulate the transfersomes. Dissodium EDTA (Sucesores de Jose Escuder, S.L., Barcelona, Spain), PEG-6 stearate (and) Ceteth-20 (and) Steareth-20 (Gattefosse España, Madrid, Spain), Cetyl Sterayl alcohol (Basf, Barcelona, Spain), medium chain triglicerides (Oximed expres S.A., Barcelona, Spain) and Xanthan gum (Azelis españa S.A., Barcelona, Spain) were used to formulate the emulsion. Metanol (Scharlab S.L., Barcelona, Spain), Nile Red, Hoeschst, phosphate buffer saline, paraformaldehyde (Sigma Aldrich, Madrid, Spain), uranyl acetate, optimal cutting temperature compound (IESMAT S.A., Barcelona, Spain), were used to perform the different analyses.

2.2. Production of Retinyl Palmitate-Loaded Transfersomes

Transfersomes were manufactured by the sonication method [22,23]. α-Tocopherol (0.02% w/w), ceramide III (0.10% w/w), phosphatydilcholine (1.78% w/w), tween 80 (0.10% w/w) and RP (1.10% w/w) were dissolved in ethanol (10% w/w) (organic phase). Then, milliQ water (qs 100% w/w) was added to the organic phase, and the system was vortexed for 1 min. Afterwards, the mixture was sonicated with a probe sonicator (amplitude of 80%, 5 min, Energy 7000 Ws, Frequency 23.88 kHz). The transfersomes' suspension was left to settle at room temperature, protected from the light. Additionally, empty transfersomes (without RP) were fabricated, to study the effect of RP on the physio-chemical characteristics of the nanosystems.

2.3. Transfersome Incorporation in a Cream Formulation

A mixture of surfactants (PEG-6 stearate (and) Ceteth-20 (and) Steareth-20 4% w/w and Cetyl Stearyl Alcohol 0.5% w/w), oils (Medium Chain Triglycerides or MCT 3% w/w) and an aqueous phase (12.6% w/w) with Xanthan gum (0.1% w/w) and disodium EDTA (0.1% w/w) were warmed up separately at 70–80 °C in a thermostatic bath. Once both phases were heated, the oil phase was added to the aqueous phase under mechanical stirring at 15,000 rpm for 2 min (Ultra-Turrax IKA T25, disperser unit S25KD 25F), and the mixture was allowed to cool down at 30 °C. Then, the transfersomes aqueous suspension, with RP at a concentration of 1.1% w/w, was added to the cream at a ratio of 1:1, so that the final RP concentration was 0.55% w/w (chosen taking the recommended concentrations for Retinol and Retinyl palmitate into account [5]). For the manufacture of the non-transfersomes emulsion, water was added up to 100%.

2.4. Transfersomes Physic-Chemical Characterization

RP-loaded transfersomes were subjected to a stability study in 25 ± 2 °C/60% ± 5% RH and 40 ± 2 °C/75% ± 5% RH chambers for 18 and 6 months, respectively, and conditioned in hermetically sealed glass vials.

Hydrodynamic size, polydispersion index (PDI) and zeta potential were studied through dynamic light scattering (DLS) using a Zetasizer Nano ZS (Malvern, UK). Dilutions of 1:10 in water were used for the measurements.

Transfersome morphology was studied through transmission electron microscopy (TEM) using a Jeol JEM 1010 100 kv (Jeol, Tokyo, Japan). TEM grids were coated with formvar of a 1:10 transfersome dilution in milliQ water and incubated for 1 min at room temperature. Grids were then washed with water and stained with a 2% w/w uranyl acetate solution for 1 min at room temperature. Afterwards, they were dried in overnight and analyzed within two weeks of staining.

The flexibility of the transfersomes was analyzed by extruding the transfersomes solution in an Avanti Mini Extruder with a 100 nm pore size polycarbonate membrane, at 1 mL of volume capacity. Pressure was applied by hand. The ability of the transfersomes to recover their initial size after extrusion was analyzed though DLS. The deformability index (DI) was defined as Equation (1),

$$DI = \left(\frac{r_p}{r_m}\right)^2 \quad (1)$$

where r_p is the radius of a the extruded transfersomes and r_m is the radius of the membrane pores [24].

2.5. Cream Physic-Chemical Characterization

Appearance (visual observation), pH (pHmeter Crison Instruments S.A. Alella, Spain) and viscosity (Brookfield RDV-III Ultra, Spain. Spindler: SC4-21, Speed: 200 rpm, Temperature: 25 °C, Spain) were studied for the transfersome- and non-transfersome-loaded emulsions.

2.6. Diffusion Assay of RP-Loaded Transfersomes

In vitro diffusion of free RP and RP from the transfersomes ($n = 6$) was studied using vertical Franz Cells (VidraFoc, Spain, receptor compartment of 12 mL, diffusional area of 2.54 cm^2). MCT was used as a receptor medium (RM) to keep sink conditions along the experiment. The dose of each formulation tested in the donor compartment was 240 mg (1.04 mg/cm^2). The temperature of the experiment was maintained at 32 °C, and the stirring speed of the RM was 500 rpm. The membrane used was Polyvinylidne Fluoride (PVDF, Millipore, Spain) of a pore diameter 0.22 µm.

Aliquots of 300 µL were taken at times 1, 2, 3, 4, 6, 24 and 30 h and injected into HPLC to quantify the amount of diffused RP.

2.7. RP HPLC Analysis and Encapsulation Efficiency

The encapsulation efficiency (% EE) of RP in the liposomes was determined indirectly (Equation (2)). Briefly, transfersomes were centrifuged in 30 KDa Amicon ultracentrifugal filter (Merck Millipore) at 4500 rpm for 30 min. The amount of RP in the filtrate and in transfersomes were analyzed using a HPLC (Waters 2695, Spain), with a photodiode array detector (Waters 2996, Spain) with the corresponding calibration curve (Range 3.40 to 280 µg/mL with an r^2 > 0.999). The column was a C18 (12.5 × 4.6 mm) with particle size of 5 µm. The mobile phase was an isocratic mixture of Metanol:water (98:2). The flow rate was 1.8 mL/min and the injection volume was 20 µL. the samples' temperature was set at 5 °C and column temperature at 40 °C. % EE was determined using Equation (2),

$$\% EE = \frac{W_{NE} - W_T}{W_T} \times 100 \quad (2)$$

where W_{NE} is the amount of RP quantified in the filtrate (RP not encapsulated) and W_T is the RP quantified in the total amount of RP used for the preparation of transfersomes.

2.8. Pig Skin Penetration Assays

Three to four month old male and female pigs were obtained from the Animal Facility at Bellvitge Campus of Barcelona University (Barcelona, Spain). Immediately after the animals ($n = 3$) were sacrificed, using an overdose of sodium thiopental anesthesia, the ears were surgically removed and frozen. On the day of experiment, ears were defrosted and the skin was excised.

2.8.1. Skin Penetration Assay: Full Thickness Pig Ear Skin

Skin samples were mounted on Franz-cells ($n = 6$) according to the description in Section 2.6. The following formulations were tested: RP-loaded transfersomes, a free RP solution in MCT, transfersome-loaded emulsion (T emulsion) and a non-encapsulated RP emulsion. An amount of 240 mg of formula was administered in infinite doses in non-occluded conditions.

After 24 h, RP mass-balance was performed: RM was analyzed directly by mean HPLC, then the non-penetrated formulation in the donor compartment (non-penetrated) was recovered and RP was extracted from the emulsion according to the method described in Section 2.7. Skin pieces were taken and washed with distilled water (wash), and stratum corneum, epidermis and dermis were obtained, and RP extracted according to the methodology described in Section 2.8.2 and analyzed by HPLC [25,26].

2.8.2. Skin Layers Recovery

An incubation solution of RP in receptor medium at a concentration of 0.22 mg/mL was prepared, then skin layers were separated and incubated for 24 h with the incubation solution. After incubation, an extraction process was performed. Skin samples were subjected to 20 min of bath sonication in Metanol:water (98:2) and RP from the different skin layers was quantified by means of HPLC (Section 2.7). Stratum corneum was removed by applying 30 tape strips (pressure 225 g/cm^2 for three seconds [27]). To separate epidermis and dermis, samples (after stripping) were immersed in 60 °C PBS for 2 min and excised with the help of forceps and a scalpel. The recovery percentage was applied to the results obtained in the penetration assays.

$$\% \ Recovery = \frac{\frac{Qextracted}{Sample\ mass}}{\frac{(Q0h - Q24h)}{Sample\ mass}} \times 100 \qquad (3)$$

The percentage of recovery was calculated from Equation (3), where "Qextracted" is the amount of RP extracted from the sample after solvent incubation (Metanol:Water 98:2), "Q0h" is the initial amount of RP in the incubation solution at time 0, "Q24h" is the amount of RP in the incubation formula after 24 h of experiment and "Sample mass" is the mass of each skin layer sample. RP analyses were performed according to Section 2.7.

2.9. Fluorescence Biodistribution Assay

To study the biodistribution of the transfersomes in the skin, fluorescent-marked transfersomes were incubated on top of full-thickness ear pig skin samples using vertical Franz Cells (according to Section 2.8.1). Non-loaded transfersomes (autofluorescence control), Nile red-loaded transfersomes and free Nile red solution were added to the experiment (all at concentrations of 0.312 μg/mL).

After 24 h of incubation, skin samples were taken and cut into 0.25 cm^2 pieces. They were then fixed with 4% paraformaldehyde (PF) for 30 min. Then, samples were washed with a phosphate buffer solution (PBS), and incubated in increasing concentrations of sucrose (up to 30% *w/w*) as a cryoprotectant. Samples were mounted in an optimal cutting temperature compound (OCT, from Fischer Scientific) and cut in the cryostat (Leica Biosystems) with a thickness between 30 and 50 μm, and placed on the superfrost slides with poly-lysine coating.

The slides were washed with PBS to remove the remaining OCT and incubated with Hoeschst (2 μg/mL) for 30 min, and then washed with PBS. Samples were visualized by a Leica DMIRB Wide Field Fluorescence and Transmitted Light Microscope [28].

2.10. TEWL after In Vivo Topical Administration

An in vivo test was carried out in humans with T and NT emulsion. The study was conducted according to the Declaration of Helsinki. Volunteers gave their written consent. Transepidermal water loss (TEWL) was measured by the Vapometer (Delfin Technologies, Kuopio, Finland) before and after the application of the different creams to monitor SC removal [29]. A template with three application zones (NT emulsion, T emulsion and negative control: no emulsion applied) with an area of 2.54 cm^2 for the forearm was used.

Six male and female individuals (n = 6) with ages ranging from 23 to 44 years old participated. An amount of 0.025 g of each emulsion was applied on the skin by the same operator in the same conditions. After 2 h, skin was gently cleaned [30].

3. Results and Discussion

3.1. Transfersomes Physico-Chemical Characterization

The manufacture of empty liposomes (without RP) was unsuccessful. During the cooling process after sonication, the viscosity of the formula increased greatly, forming a gel, and no transfersomes were formed.

The RP-loaded transfersomes obtained had a hydrodynamic diameter of 300.5 nm with PDI = 0.471, and a negative charge (Table 1). The % EE of RP was quantified by HPLC, as 100%. The RP limit of detection (LOD) and limit of quantification (LOQ) of the analytical method were 0.22 and 0.72 µg/mL, calculated by the signal to noise ratio). No RP was observed in the filtrate, demonstrating that all had been encapsulated. This fact, and the increased viscosity in empty transfersomes, seems to indicate that the entire RP is integrated with the transfersome membrane, and its presence is essential for the correct stabilization and formation of the nanosystems.

Table 1. Transfersome physical chemical parameters, measured by dynamic light scattering (DLS) and HPLC. Assay (%) refers to the HPLC retinyl palmitate (RP) quantification assay respect to the nominal value of RP (1.1% w/w).

Sample	Hydrodynamic Diameter (nm)	PDI	Z-Potential (mv)	Assay (%)	EE (%)
Transfersomes	300.5 ± 10.9	0.471 ± 0.020	−9.48 ± 1.50	102.63 ± 0.51	100 ± 0

Transfersomes had a spherical shape (Figure 1). Mean particle diameter was also measured by TEM to corroborate the size results obtained in DLS with the TEM images, and to study the morphology of the vesicles. Using Image J software, the diameter obtained was 238.48 ± 29.74 nm. The fact that the diameter obtained in TEM is smaller than in DLS is due to the solvation of the transfersomes when measured in aqueous suspension.

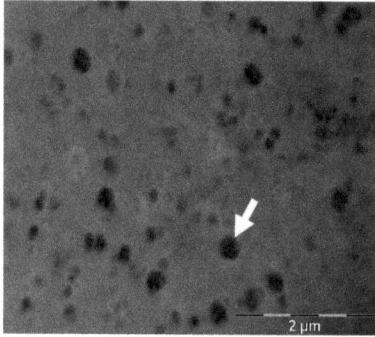

Figure 1. Transmission electron microscopy pictures of negative-stained transfersomes with uranyl acetate.

After manufacturing, transfersomes were stored in climate chambers at 25 °C/60% HR for 18 months and 40 °C/75% HR for six months (as accelerated conditions). Regression analysis of particle size and PDI was performed to check their evolution over time (Figures 2 and 3). As can be seen in

Table 2, the slope's p-values were above 0.05, so the regression lines are statistically equal to zero, which means the RP-loaded transfersomes kept their hydrodynamic diameter and PDI stable at these conditions. The lack of significant variations at accelerated conditions, according to ICH Q1E [31], means the estimated product shelf-life can be extended to 36 months.

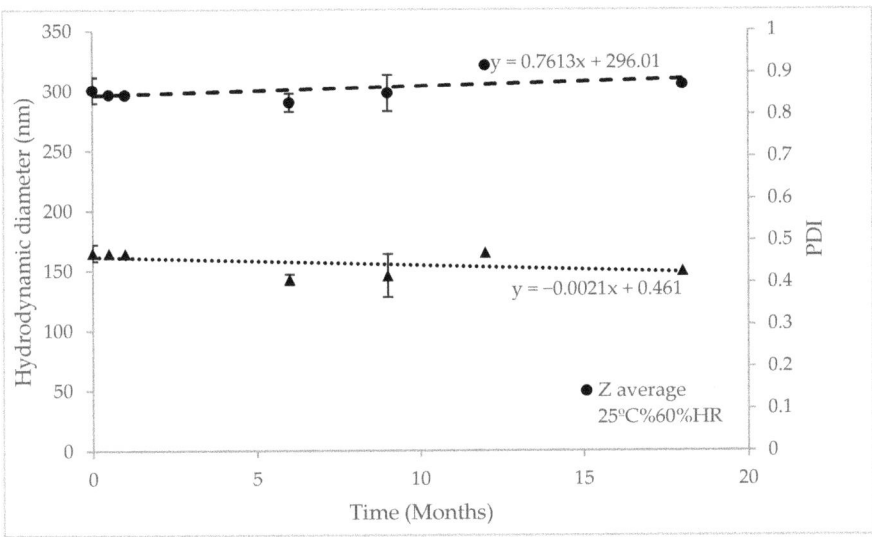

Figure 2. Stability studies at 25 ± 2 °C/60% ± 5% Relative Humidity (HR) over 18 months. RP-loaded transfersomes' hydrodynamic diameter and polydispersity index, monitored over time.

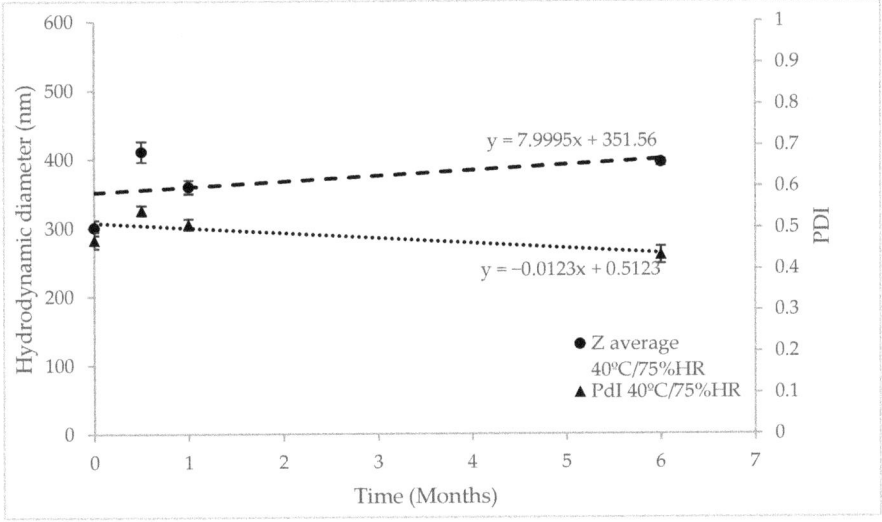

Figure 3. Stability studies at 40 ± 2 °C/75% ± 5% HR for six months. RP-loaded transfersomes' hydrodynamic diameter and polydispersity index, monitored over time.

Table 2. Transfersome stability regression slopes.

Condition	25 °C/60% HR		40 °C/75% HR	
Response	Hydrodynamic Diameter	PDI	Hydrodynamic Diameter (nm)	PDI
Slope	0.761	−0.002	8.000	−0.012
p-value	0.231	0.277	0.546	0.275

Transfersomes are defined as deformable liposomes, due to the presence of edge activators. To assess their flexibility, the Teixeira et al. method was used. This demonstrated the flexibility of their polymeric nanocapsules, based on the particles' ability to recover their initial size after extrusion [32]. On the other hand, Yu-Kyoung Oh et al. [9] studied the deformability index of transfersomes manufactured with different edge activators. They obtained the highest DI with tween80 and tween20 (DI = 6 and 8.45, respectively).

In this study, RP transfersomes were extruded by a 100 nm pore size membrane, approximately three times smaller than their hydrodynamic diameter. The vesicle size and PDI before and after extrusion is shown in Table 3, as well as the DI. The difference in diameter is very small, showing their ability to recover their size after extrusion. However, a small proportion of the particles, probably the largest, are partially extruded, which explains the PDI decrease. These results are consistent with the results obtained by Teixeira et al. These results are also in agreement with Yu-Kyoung Oh et al., as the DI results are similar when choosing polysorbates as edge activators.

Table 3. Transfersomes' diameter, polydispersion index (PDI) and deformability index.

Sample	Hydrodynamic Diameter (nm)	PDI	Deformability Index
Transfersomes	300.5 ± 10.9	0.471 ± 0.020	
Extruded Transfersomes	285.5 ± 9.7	0.247 ± 0.014	8.12

3.2. Transfersome Cream Physic-Chemical Characterization

Transfersome cream formulation and non-transfersome cream formulation appearance, pH and viscosities are shown in Table 4. The pH was in the same range as the human skin pH (between 4.5 and 5.5). Transfersome cream viscosity was higher, due to the increase in total lipid components. Both cream RP contents were assayed, and the obtained results were between 95% and 105%.

Table 4. Physio-chemical parameters of transfersome and non-transfersome cream formulations.

Sample	Appearance	pH	Viscosity (cP)	Assay (%)
NT Cream	White-yellowish cream	4.86	64.70 ± 0.18	98.07 ± 0.68
T Cream	White-yellowish cream	4.81	100.15 ± 2.35	96.87 ± 0.72

3.3. Synthetic Membrane RP Difussion Assay

Table 5 shows the % RP released at different timepoints from the transfersomes. Only 7.64% of RP was able to diffuse through the synthetic membrane after 30 h of experiment. Until six hours of experiment, no RP peak appeared in any of the chromatograms. As discussed previously, RP is completely integrated into the liposome membrane, forming a structural part of it. The presence of RP in the receptor medium at longer timepoints could be due to the drug diffusion from the liposomal lamella to the receptor medium (based on sink conditions), which is the classical release theory. However, although the membrane's pore size does not allow transferome to pass through, it demonstrated their flexibility. Due to the lack of pressure from extrusion, vesicle translocation to RM across membrane pores takes a longer time to occur. Once transfersome crosses the pore, hydrophobic solution make them destructured and causes them to release RP. To ensure that intact transfersomes were able to cross the membrane pore, the experiment was replicated with water as the receptor medium instead of MCT, because DLS characterization would not be possible in this medium. After 24 h, an aliquot was extracted and measured by DLS. A population with a similar size (approximately 280 nm) appears, even though the count rate (kcps) was low (less than 200), indicating a low concentration of particles in the sample.

Table 5. RP-released percentage through a synthetic membrane from a transfersome formulation.

Time (h)	Mean RP Released (%)	Standard Deviation (%)
4	0	0
6	0.36	0.57
24	6.81	6.19
30	7.64	6.61

3.4. Franz-Cells Full-Thickness Pig Skin Penetration Assays

3.4.1. Transfersomes' RP Penetration

Figure 4 shows the penetration profile of RP from transfersomes and control (free RP solution in MCT) formulations in the different skin layers. Mass balance ranged between 90%–110% recovery in both cases.

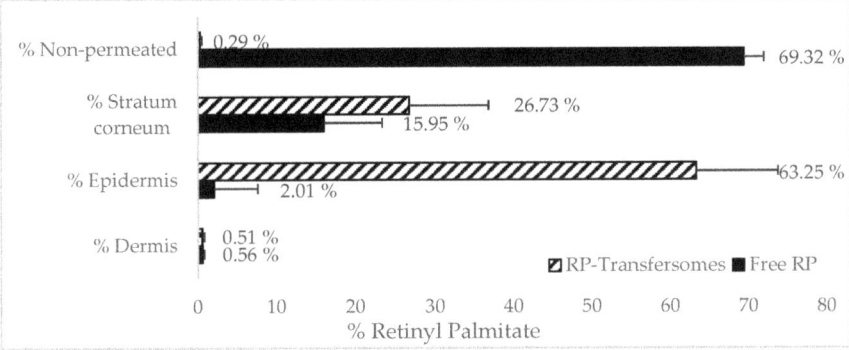

Figure 4. Black bar shows the free retinyl palmitate penetration. The black stripped bars show the RP penetration from transfersomes.

RP was not detected in the receptor medium in any of the formulations after 24 h, which seems to indicate that, after topical application, RP would not reach systemic circulation.

Vehiculation in transfersomes has a significant effect on the biodistribution of RP in the different layers of the skin. In the case of non-vehiculated RP, most of the active ingredients did not penetrate the skin (69%) and only 2% reached the epidermis. The RP logP was around 15 [5] which is far from the optimal range (2–3) [33] to obtain maximum transdermal permeability. Its molecular weight is near 500 Da, which is considered the maximum value for transdermal absorption [34]. Therefore, it is expected to have a poor permeability.

The percentage of RP found in the stratum corneum was higher in transfersomes (26%) than in free solution. Stratum corneum can act as a reservoir with a depot effect for epidermis absorption. However, part of this amount will also be eliminated during the natural desquamation cycle of the stratum corneum.

RP found in epidermis was much higher in the case of transfersomes (63%), demonstrating that the increase in the delivery of RP into epidermis results in viable keratinocytes being found, which lead to its pharmacological effect. These results confirm the promoting effect of transfersomes for RP absorption, compared with a free solution of RP. Similar results were found by Yu-Kyoung Oh et al., who demonstrated an increase in the penetration of deformable liposomes based on the tween20 encapsulating retinol [9] compared with classic liposomes and free retinol solution. An increase in the epidermal delivery of RP loaded in vesicles was also obtained by Clares et al. [35]. In a study with dermatomized skin (0.4 μm) the liposomal systems demonstrates a greater penetration of nanoemulsions and solid lipid nanoparticles. Teixeira et al. [32] performed similar penetration assays on RP loaded in polymeric nanocapsules. Both of them obtained similar results to the ones shown in this research, of an approximately three-fold increase in RP levels in deep skin layers, compared with the amount found in the stratum corneum.

3.4.2. Emulsions RP Penetration

It is very common to introduce liposomes or other topical drug delivery systems into emulsions to improve their attractiveness to final users. The inclusion of these formulations in emulsion could modify their physicochemical and biopharmaceutical characteristics. In order to evaluate the dilution effect and how the emulsification process could affect the transfersomes' properties, a manufacturing simulation was carried out, because of the difficulty of finding transfersomes inside emulsions by electronic microscopy. RP transfersome solution was heated at the emulsion oil phase melting point (70–80 °C) for 15 min, then a water phase at the same temperature was added to the transfersome solution and mixed for 2 min with mechanical stirring at 15,000 rpm with the ultraturrax. Resulted solution was allowed to cold down and, after 24 h, vesicle size and PDI were measured by DLS, obtaining transfersomes of 266.4 nm and PDI 0.554. Even though this experiment cannot prove if the transfersomes fuse with the lipid components of the cream or not, it does demonstrate that transfersomes are able to resist the dilution effect and the emulsification process.

Figure 5 shows the penetration of RP T emulsion and NT emulsion. It seems that the inclusion of transfersomes in an emulsion slows down the epidermis absorption, but, conversely, transfersomes increase the delivery of RP into epidermis. It seems that the emulsion could improve the dermis absorption of RT when transfersomes are used. In this case, the RP found in SC did not exhibit large differences between formulations. The presence of additional surfactants and emollients in the emulsion seems to improve RP disposition in SC when they are not loaded in transfersomes, but the epidermal and dermal delivery is still higher in the presence of transfersomes.

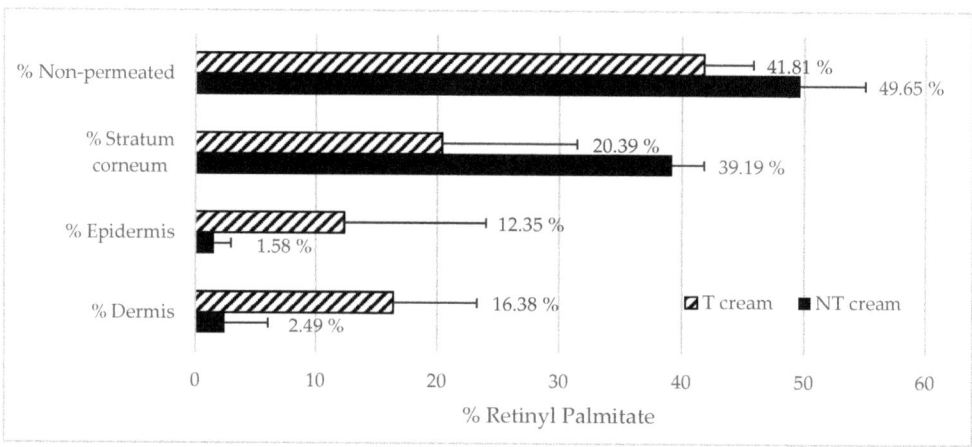

Figure 5. Black bar shows the RP penetration from Non-transfersome (NT) emulsion. The black stripped bars show the RP penetration from T emulsion.

3.5. Fluorescence Biodistribution Assay

In order to confirm the increase in the epidermal delivery of RP in transfersomes, a fluorescence microscopy experiment was carried out with Nile red-loaded transfersomes and a free Nile red solution. Figure 6 shows the superposition of two fluorescence emission measurements from the same area of the skin sample (emission in the blue range for the cell nuclei stained by Hoeschst, and red for the Nile red formulation). As can be seen, the control of Nile red free solution (Figure 6a) only shows red fluorescence in the most superficial layer of the skin (stratum corneum), while the fluorescent marker loaded in transfersomes penetrates towards inner layers of the skin and, consequently, red fluorescence is observed (Figure 6b). These results agree with the results of the quantification of RP in the different layers of the skin, in which an accumulation of active ingredients in the epidermis and dermis was observed when it was vehiculized in transfersomes.

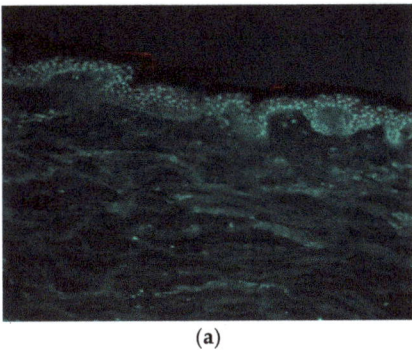
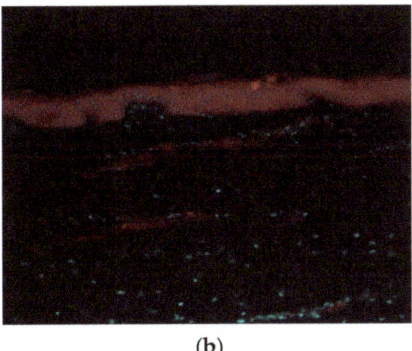

(a)   (b)

Figure 6. Fluorescence microscopy images of pig-ear skin cross-section. Red color corresponds to Nile red fluorescence and blue to Hoeschst staining of the cell nucleus. (**a**) Not vehiculized nile red control (image J, mean epidermis intensity 7846 ± 140 AU); (**b**) Nile red-marked transfersomes (image J, mean epidermis intensity 12,428 ± 254 AU). The images were captured using 10× magnifications

3.6. In Vivo Topical RP Penetration

The T and NT emulsions were tested in six volunteers for the screening of skin compatibility (based on TEWL measurement) and for RP quantification in the stratum corneum. Table 6 shows the TEWL (g/m^2 h) measurements for each individual before and after application of the formulations. In order to study the stability of TEWL measurements, a t-test between the TEWL ratio and one was performed before and after application. No statistical differences were found, which means that the integrity of the skin is not affected by the formulations.

Table 6. Transepidermal water loss (TEWL) average measures before and after the application of L and NT creams, as well as p value of the comparation between the ratio and 1 before and after application.

Time 0 h TEWL (g/m^2 h)	Standard Deviation (g/m^2 h)	Time 2 h after Application TWEL (g/m^2 h)	Standard Deviation (g/m^2 h)	Ratio TWEL 2 h/0 h	p-Value vs. 1
11.17	1.25	10.63	0.99	0.95	0.388

Two hours after application, the skin surface was cleaned, and tape strips were taken from each individual until TEWL values increased to 30–35 g/m^2 h. A two sample t-test was performed to analyze the significance of the differences between the ratio and 1 before and after application, and there were no significative differences, as can be seen in Table 4 (p value 0.388).

4. Conclusions

Deformable transfersomes were successfully obtained with RP, integrated in the liposome membrane, with an estimated shelf-life of 36 months. RP-loaded transfersomes demonstrated an increase in penetration into the skin layers under the stratum corneum of the skin in vitro compared to a free RP control. Similarly, the inclusion of transfersomes to an emulsion increased RP skin penetration compared to the same emulsion without transfersomes. These results are reinforced thanks to the biodistribution experiment with fluorescence microscopy, where a significant increase in epidermis penetration was observed. The in vivo study demonstrated the compatibility of the tested formulations. Given these results, the developed transfersome formulation is a good candidate to increase the delivery of highly lipophilic drugs such as RP to the epidermis.

Author Contributions: F.F.-C. conceived and designed this study and revised the manuscript; E.P.-R. and M.C.M. performed the studies; B.B.-F. participated in the performance of these studies; E.P.-R. analyzed the data, created the graphics and wrote the paper; J.G. provided funding acquisition and supervised this project. All authors have read and agreed to the published version of the manuscript.

Funding: This research received no external funding.

Acknowledgments: Assistance provided by Manel Bosch and Marta Taulés from the University of Barcelona Scientific-Technical service was greatly appreciated.

Conflicts of Interest: The authors declare no conflict of interest.

References

1. Gerard, J.; James, G.; Mezick, A. Pharmacological effects of retinoids on skin cells. *Ski. Pharm.* **1993**, *6*, 24–34.
2. Mukherjee, S.; Date, A.; Patravale, V.; Korting, H.C.; Roeder, A.; Weindl, G. Retinoids in the treatment of skin aging: An overview of clinical efficacy and safety. *Clin. Interv. Aging.* **2006**, *1*, 327–348. [CrossRef] [PubMed]
3. Jean, J.; Soucy, J.; Roxane, P. Effects of Retinoic Acid on Keratinocyte Proliferation and Differentiation in a Psoriatic Skin Model. *Tissue Eng. Part A* **2011**, *17*, 13–14. [CrossRef] [PubMed]
4. O'Byrne, S.M.; Blaner, W.S. Retinol and retinyl esters: Biochemistry and physiology. *J. Lipid Res.* **2013**, *54*, 1731–1743. [CrossRef] [PubMed]
5. Scientific Committee on Consumer Safety. *Opinion on Vitamin A (Retinol, Retinyl Acetate, Retinyl Palmitate)*; Scientific Committee on Consumer Safety: Brussels, Belgium, 2016.
6. MacGregor, J.L.; Maibach, H.I. The Specificity of Retinoid-Induced Irritation and Its Role in Clinical Efficacy. *Exog. Dermatol.* **2002**, *1*, 68–73. [CrossRef]
7. Kim, B.H.; Lee, Y.S.; Kang, K.S. The mechanism of retinol-induced irritation and its application to anti-irritant development. *Toxicol. Lett.* **2003**, *146*, 65–73. [CrossRef]
8. Liu, J.C.; Wang, J.C.T.; Yusuf, M.; Yamamoto, N.; Kazama, S.; Stahl, C.R.; Holland, J.P.; Mather, K.; Aleles, M.A.; Hamada, S.; et al. Topical Oil in Water Emulsions Containing Retinoids. U.S. Patent No. 5976555, 2 November 1999.
9. Oh, Y.; Kim, M.Y.; Shin, J.; Kim, T.W.; Yun, M.; Yang, S.J.; Choi, S.S.; Jung, W.; Kim, J.A.; Choi, H. Skin permeation of retinol in Tween 20-based deformable liposomes: In-vitro evaluation in human skin and keratinocyte models. *J. Pharm. Pharmacol.* **2006**, *58*, 161–166. [CrossRef]
10. Bozzuto, G.; Molinari, A. Liposomes as nanomedical devices. *Int. J. Nanomed.* **2015**, *10*, 975–999. [CrossRef]
11. Braun-Falco, O.; Kortung, H.C.; Maibach, H.I. (Eds.) *Griesb Ach Conference: Liposomes Dermatics*; Springer: Berlin/Heidelberg, Germany, 1992.
12. Touitou, E.; Dayan, N.; Bergelson, L.; Godin, B.; Eliaz, M. Ethosomes–novel vesicular carriers for enhanced delivery: Characterization and skin penetration properties. *J. Control. Release* **2000**, *65*, 403–418. [CrossRef]
13. Jain, S.; Jain, P.; Umamaheshwari, R.B.; Jain, N.K. Transfersomes—A Novel Vesicular Carrier for Enhanced Transdermal Delivery: Development, Characterization, and Performance Evaluation. *Drug Dev. Ind. Pharm.* **2003**, *29*, 1013–1026. [CrossRef]

14. Paul, A.; Cevc, G.; Bachhawat, B.K. Transdermal immunization with an integral membrane component gap junction protein, by means of ultradeformable drug carriers, transfersomes. *Vaccine* **1998**, *16*, 188–195. [CrossRef]
15. Cevc, G. Transfersomes, liposomes and other lipid suspension on the skin, permeation enhancement, vesicles penetration and transdermal drug delivery. *Crit. Rev. Ther. Drug Carr. Syst.* **1996**, *13*, 257–388. [CrossRef] [PubMed]
16. Omar, M.M.; Hasan, O.A.; El Sisi, A.M. Preparation and optimization of lidocaine transferosomal gel containing permeation enhancers: A promising approach for enhancement of skin permeation. *Int. J. Nanomed.* **2019**, *14*, 1551–1562. [CrossRef] [PubMed]
17. Coderch, L.; López, O.; de la Maza, A.; Parra, J.L. Ceramides and skin function. *Am. J. Clin. Dermatol.* **2003**, *4*, 107–129. [CrossRef]
18. Motta, S.; Sesana, S.; Monti, M.; Giuliani, A.; Caputo, R. Interlamellar lipid differences between normal and psoriatic stratum corneum. *Acta Derm. Venereologica. Suppl.* **1994**, *186*, 131–132.
19. Matsumoto, N.U.M. Difference in Ceramide Composition between "Dry" and "Normal" Skin in Patients with Atopic Dermatitis. *Acta Derm. Venereol.* **1999**, *79*, 246–247. [CrossRef]
20. Barbosa-Barros, L.; de la Maza, A.; López-Iglesias, C.; López, O. Ceramide effects in the bicelle structure. *Colloids Surf. A Physicochem. Eng. Asp.* **2008**, *317*, 576–584. [CrossRef]
21. Shabbits, J.A.; Mayer, L.D. Intracellular delivery of ceramide lipids via liposomes enhances apoptosis in vitro. *Biochim. Biophys. Acta (BBA) Biomembr.* **2003**, *1612*, 98–106. [CrossRef]
22. Woodbury, D.J.; Richardson, E.S.; Grigg, A.W.; Welling, R.D.; Knudson, B.H. Reducing Liposome Size with Ultrasound: Bimodal Size Distributions. *J. Liposome Res.* **2006**, *16*, 57–80. [CrossRef]
23. Jesorka, A.; Orwar, O. Liposomes: Technologies and Analytical Applications. *Annu. Rev. Anal. Chem.* **2008**, *1*, 801–832. [CrossRef]
24. Cevc, G.; Gebauer, D.; Stieber, J.; Schätzlein, A.; Blume, G. Ultraflexible vesicles, Transfersomes, have an extremely low pore penetration resistance and transport therapeutic amounts of insulin across the intact mammalian skin. *Biochim. Et Biophys. Acta (BBA) Biomembr.* **1998**, *1368*, 201–215. [CrossRef]
25. European Centre for the Validation of Alternative Methods (CVAM). *Test Guideline for Skin Absorption: In Vitro Method*; Official Journal of the European Union Method B.45 of Annex to 440/2008/EC; European Commission: Paris, France, 2008.
26. Nangia, A.; Berner, B.; Maibach, H.I. *Transepidermal Water Loss Measurements for Assessing Skin Barrier Functions During in vitro Percutaneous Absorption Studies*; Bronaugh, R.L., Maibach, H.I., Eds.; Percutaneous Absorption Drugs, Cosmetics, Mechanisms Methodology, Drugs and the Pharmaceutical Sciences, Marcel Dekker Inc.: New York, NY, USA, 1999; pp. 587–594.
27. Dabboue, H.; Builles, N.; Frouin, E.; Scott, D.; Ramos, J.; Marti-Mestres, G. Assessing the Impact of Mechanical Damage on Full-Thickness Porcine and Human Skin Using an In Vitro Approach. *BioMed Res. Int.* **2015**, *2015*, 1–10. [CrossRef]
28. Wilhelm, K.P.; Elsner, P.; Berardesca, E.; Maibach, H.I. *Bioengineering of the Skin: Skin Imaging and Analysis*, 2nd ed.; CRC Press: Boca Raton, FL, USA, 1996.
29. Elmahjoubi, E.; Frum, Y.; Eccleston, G.M.; Wilkinson, S.C.; Meidan, V.M. Transepidermal water loss for probing full-thickness skin barrier function: Correlation with tritiated water flux, sensitivity to punctures and diverse surfactant exposures. *Toxicol. Vitr.* **2009**, *23*, 1429–1435. [CrossRef] [PubMed]
30. Klang, V.; Schwarz, J.C.; Lenobel, B.; Nadj, M.; Auböck, J.; Wolzt, M.; Valenta, C. In vitro vs. in vivo tape stripping: Validation of the porcine ear model and penetration assessment of novel sucrose stearate emulsions. *Eur. J. Pharm. Biopharm.* **2012**, *80*, 604–614. [CrossRef] [PubMed]
31. Baber, N. International conference on harmorisation of technical requirements for registration of pharmaceutical for human use. *Br. J. Clin. Pharmacol.* **1994**, *37*, 401–404. [CrossRef] [PubMed]
32. Teixeira, Z.; Zanchetta, B.; Melo, B.A.; Oliveira, L.L.; Santana, M.H.; Paredes-Gamero, E.J.; Justo, G.Z.; Nader, H.B.; Guterres, S.S.; Durán, N. Retinyl palmitate flexible polymeric nanocapsules: Characterization and permeation studies. *Colloids Surf. B Biointerfaces* **2010**, *81*, 374–380. [CrossRef] [PubMed]
33. Benson, H.A.E.; Warkinson, A.C. *Transdermal and Topical Drug Delivery, Principles and Practice*; John Wiley & Sons, Inc.: Hoboken, NJ, USA, 2011; Chapter 1; p. 17.

34. Singh, I.; Morris, A.P. Performance of transdermal therapeutic systems: Effects of biological factors. *Int. J. Pharm. Investig.* **2011**, *1*, 4–9. [CrossRef]
35. Clares, B.; Calpena, A.C.; Parra, A.; Abrego, G.; Alvarado, H.; Fangueiro, J.F.; Souto, E.B. Nanoemulsions (NEs), liposomes (LPs) and solid lipid nanoparticles (SLNs) for retinyl palmitate: Effect on skin permeation. *Int. J. Pharm.* **2014**, *473*, 591–598. [CrossRef]

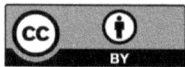

© 2020 by the authors. Licensee MDPI, Basel, Switzerland. This article is an open access article distributed under the terms and conditions of the Creative Commons Attribution (CC BY) license (http://creativecommons.org/licenses/by/4.0/).

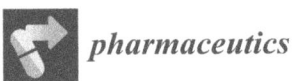

Article

Endogenous Antioxidant Cocktail Loaded Hydrogel for Topical Wound Healing of Burns

José L. Soriano [1], Ana C. Calpena [2,3,*], María J. Rodríguez-Lagunas [4,5], Òscar Domènech [2,3], Nuria Bozal-de Febrer [6], María L. Garduño-Ramírez [7] and Beatriz Clares [1,3,8,*]

1. Department of Pharmacy and Pharmaceutical Technology, Faculty of Pharmacy, University of Granada, 18071 Granada, Spain; jlsoriano@correo.ugr.es
2. Department of Pharmacy and Pharmaceutical Technology and Physical Chemistry, Faculty of Pharmacy and Food Sciences, University of Barcelona, 08028 Barcelona, Spain; odomenech@ub.edu
3. Nanoscience & Nanotechnology Institute (IN2UB), University of Barcelona, 08028 Barcelona, Spain
4. Department of Biochemistry and Physiology, Faculty of Pharmacy and Food Sciences, University of Barcelona, 08028 Barcelona, Spain; mjrodriguez@ub.edu
5. Nutrition and Food Safety Research Institute (INSA-UB), 08921 Santa Coloma de Gramenet, Spain
6. Department of Biology, Healthcare and the Environment, Faculty of Pharmacy and Food Sciences, University of Barcelona, 27-31 Joan XXIII Ave., 08028 Barcelona, Spain; nuriabozaldefebrer@ub.edu
7. Centro de Investigaciones Químicas, Universidad Autónoma del Estado de Morelos, Av. Universidad No. 1001, Col Chamilpa, 62209 Cuernavaca, Mexico; lgarduno@ciq.uaem.mx
8. Biosanitary Institute of Granada (ibs.GRANADA), 18012 Granada, Spain
* Correspondence: anacalpena@ub.edu (A.C.C.); beatrizclares@ugr.es (B.C.); Tel.: +34-934-024-560 (A.C.C.); +34-958-246-664 (B.C.)

Citation: Endogenous Antioxidant Cocktail Loaded Hydrogel for Topical Wound Healing of Burns. *Pharmaceutics* 2020, 13, 8. https://dx.doi.org/10.3390/pharmaceutics13010008

Received: 26 November 2020
Accepted: 17 December 2020
Published: 22 December 2020

Publisher's Note: MDPI stays neutral with regard to jurisdictional claims in published maps and institutional affiliations.

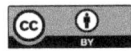

Copyright: © 2020 by the authors. Licensee MDPI, Basel, Switzerland. This article is an open access article distributed under the terms and conditions of the Creative Commons Attribution (CC BY) license (https://creativecommons.org/licenses/by/4.0/).

Abstract: The main goal of this work is the study of the skin wound healing efficacy of an antioxidant cocktail consisting of vitamins A, D, E and the endogenous pineal hormone melatonin (MLT), with all of these loaded into a thermosensitive hydrogel delivery system. The resulting formulation was characterized by scanning electron microscopy. The antioxidant efficacy and microbiological activity against Gram positive and Gram negative strains were also assayed. The skin healing efficacy was tested using an in vivo model which included histological evaluation. Furthermore, atomic force microscopy was employed to evaluate the wound healing efficacy of rat skin burns through the determination of its elasticity at the nanoscale using force spectroscopy analysis. The resulting hydrogel exhibited sol state at low temperature and turned into a gel at 30 ± 0.2 °C. The hydrogel containing the antioxidant cocktail showed higher scavenging activity than the hydrogel containing vitamins or MLT, separately. The formulation showed optimal antimicrobial activity. It was comparable to a commercial reference. It was also evidenced that the hydrogel containing the antioxidant cocktail exhibited the strongest healing process in the skin burns of rats, similar to the assayed commercial reference containing silver sulfadiazine. Histological studies confirmed the observed results. Finally, atomic force microscopy demonstrated a similar distribution of Young's modulus values between burned skin treated with the commercial reference and burned skin treated with hydrogel containing the antioxidant cocktail, and all these with healthy skin. The use of an antioxidant cocktail of vitamins and MLT might be a promising treatment for skin wounds for future clinical studies.

Keywords: vitamins; melatonin; antioxidant; skin; healing; ATF microscopy

1. Introduction

The skin is a microbiological, chemical, immunological and physical barrier that confers protection to the organism against external harms [1]. This barrier can be disrupted, allowing external pathogens to enter the body, which causes inflammation and infection. Among skin wounds, burns are the most frequent skin injuries. This kind of injury can be caused by thermal, electrical, chemical, or electromagnetic energy. The severity of the burn correlates with the layers of the epidermis, dermis and hypodermis affected, increasing the morbidity and mortality when the surface area of the burn increases [2]. The induced damage is accompanied by the activation of inflammatory and coagulation processes, as well as an excess of cytotoxic reactive oxygen and nitrogen species (ROS, RNS), involving secondary tissue damage [3]. In this regard, the development of effective antioxidant tools for cutaneous wound healing would help to reduce tissue damage and wound infection, as well as other associated complications [4]. Recently, this antioxidant strategy has been also investigated [5,6]. Classical treatments of topical wound burns include the gold standard silver sulfadiazine. However, some detrimental effects such as cytotoxic activity and wound healing delay have been described [7]. Thus, the research of new approaches for controlling infection and avoiding undesired cytotoxic effects, at the same time, represents a challenge of paramount importance nowadays. Among antioxidant agents for wound healing, several types of vitamins have been proposed, such as vitamins E (alpha tocopherol) and D. Alpha tocopherol prevents the oxidation damage of collagen and glycosaminoglycans during wound healing, being able to accelerate the wound closure and ameliorate burn infection [8,9]. Regarding vitamin D, this vitamin has been reported to modulate immune responses [10], and it has also been proved to present a beneficial effect in sun burns [11]. Moreover, vitamin D triggers the formation of antimicrobial peptides that may contribute to the wound healing process [12]. Vitamin A, despite not being a common antioxidant, is able to reduce oxidative stress [13] and even prevent the cancer risks of oxidative damage [14]. Recent studies have shown that vitamin A favors superoxide dismutase and glutathione transferase activities [15]. Furthermore, it has also been associated with participation in wound healing, specifically in macrophage-mediated inflammatory processes as well as angiogenesis [16]. Taking all these vitamins together, we have previously developed a thermosensitive hydrogel loaded with vitamin A, D and E for the treatment of skin burns [17].

Other antioxidant molecules, such as the endogenous hormone melatonin (MLT; 5-methoxy-N-acetyl-tryptamine), has also been assayed in this field [18]. MLT is secreted by the pineal gland and plays an important role as a potent radical scavenger of reactive oxygen species (ROS) and reactive nitrogen species (RNS). In a previous paper, we reviewed the role of melatonin (MLT) as a powerful antioxidant [19]. The antioxidant effects of MLT occur through direct and indirect mechanisms. On one hand, MLT scavenges free radicals in all compartments of the body due to its amphiphilia and its distribution capacity [20]. MLT has been shown to detoxify up to 10 radicals [21]. On the other hand, MLT increases the activity of antioxidant enzymes. This causes an increase in the endogenous antioxidant defense capacity and induces the upregulation of gene expression, increasing the first line of defense against oxidative damage to cells [22]. Due to these properties, it has been proposed as a potential treatment for wound healing [23,24], being more effective than vitamins C and E [25,26]. In addition to the anti-inflammatory effect of MLT, it has some advantages with respect to other antioxidant molecules, such as its endogenous nature and its facility to enter into subcellular compartments, among others [19,27]. Among the beneficial effects of MLT, in vitro and in vivo antimicrobial properties have been also reported [28,29]. In this sense, MLT has shown activity against fungi such as *Sacchoramyces cerevisae* or *Candida albicans* [30], some viruses [31] and both Gram positive and Gram negative bacteria. Some authors have concluded that its antimicrobial activity could be due to the reduction in intracellular substrates, which leads to a prolongation of the lag phase of bacterial growth [32].

Thus, the possibility of using vitamins and MLT together might be a suitable combination for treating skin burns and improving the proliferation and differentiation of skin cells. For this task, a drug-delivery system for skin wound healing able to absorb wound exudates and provide a moist environment with intrinsic antimicrobial properties should be desirable. Different drug-delivery systems for loading these antioxidant drugs have been developed so far for treating wounds, such as microspheres [33], nanoparticles [34], nanospheres [35], etc. It is also remarkable to take into consideration the biological properties of biomaterials forming the drug carrier. In previous studies, our group has demonstrated the potential of a hydrogel loading antioxidant actives in wound healing, consisting of poloxamer 407 (PLX), chitosan (CS) and hyaluronic acid (HA) [17,36]. Hydrogel might absorb exudates and provide a moist environment, preventing wound dehydration [37]. In this context, in situ gel-forming hydrogel is even more appropriate due to its ability to fill the wound area as sol state just after topical administration and adhere when converted into gel [38].

As a next step, it is our intention to evaluate the effect of antioxidant actives, vitamins and MLT together, as well as the use of techniques that help to record the healing action of these antioxidant drugs on the skin.

Atomic Force Microscopy (AFM) has emerged as a useful technique not only to visualize samples at a nanometric level, but also as a powerful technique to quantify functional and structural characteristics from the nanoscale to the microscale, from single molecules to whole cells and tissues. AFM has been widely used to investigate individual cells [39] or the extracellular matrix (ECM) of soft tissues [40,41]. In recent years, the investigation of the whole tissue [42,43] is an emerging field to understand, in a bottom-up way, the classical biological experiments on tissues.

In the present work, we proposed a strategy for the wound healing of burns, which combined antioxidant vitamins A, E, D and the endogenous hormone MLT. The antioxidant cocktail was loaded in a PLX/CS/HA hydrogel. For this task, the wound healing efficacy was assessed in vivo and histologically. Furthermore, we evaluated the elastic modulus, Young's modulus, by means of force spectroscopy AFM (FS-AFM) of burned rat skin samples after different treatments to investigate the therapeutic goodness on a cutaneous wound model. In order to support the previous tests, the antibacterial and antioxidant activity was also determined.

2. Materials and Methods

2.1. Materials and Animals

MLT and sodium hyaluronate (1.46 MDa) were purchased from Acofar (Madrid, Spain). Retinol palmitate (vitamin A) 200,000 IU/mL, cholecalciferol (vitamin D3) 100,000 IU/g, and D,L alpha tocopherol acetate (vitamin E) were supplied by Fagron Iberica (Barcelona, Spain). PLX was obtained from BASF (Barcelona, Spain). Sigma-Aldrich (Madrid, Spain) supplied 75–85% deacetylated CS (190–310 KDa).

The commercial topical cream silvederma® containing silver sulfadiazine 10 mg/g (Aldo-Union Co., Barcelona, Spain) expiry date 01/2021, batch 0012M003, was purchased from a local pharmacy. Double distilled water was obtained from a device Milli-Q® Gradient A10 (Millipore Iberica, Madrid, Spain). All other materials used in experimental sections were of analytical grade and supplied by Sigma-Aldrich (Madrid, Spain) unless otherwise specified.

Wistar rats, 3–5 months old and weighing 300–500 g, were purchased from the Laboratory Animal Center of Barcelona University. The animals were maintained under standard conditions with free access to food and water in the laboratory animal facilities for one week before the beginning of studies. All rats were treated humanely and under veterinary supervision throughout the experimental period.

2.2. Preparation and Characterization of Hydrogel

The PLX/CS/HA based hydrogel was prepared via wet conventional synthesis by direct dispersion in water. Briefly, 0.2% HA solution (w/v) was prepared by adding the required amount of HA to double distilled water and then stirred for 1 h, subsequently the solution was filtered. Then, a 0.5 % (w/v) CS/acetic acid solution was obtained by dispersing the correct amount of CS in 0.5% acetic acid. Equally, 1.8% PLX (w/v) was dissolved in double distilled water with continuous stirring. The inclusion of actives was carried out as follows.

A pre-selected amount of vitamin D was poured into the required volumes of vitamins A and E and dispersed. This mixture, together with the amount of MLT required to reach 1% (w/v), was added to the previous PLX solution until solubilization at 4 °C. Afterwards, this solution containing actives and the CS solution were added to the HA solution at 4 °C and stirred continuously for 24 h. Finally, the required amount of PLX to reach 18% (w/v) was added, and this was left to stand for 24 h. The final composition of the formulation labeled as PLX/CS/HA-VM was: PLX 18% (w/v), CS 0.5% (w/v), HA 0.2% (w/v), vitamin A 6000 IU/g, vitamin D 400 IU/g, vitamin E 2% (w/v) and MLT 1% (w/v). Furthermore, PLX/CS/HA hydrogel loading vitamins (PLX/CS/HA-V) or MLT (PLX/CS/HA-M) were also prepared for antioxidant, histological and AFM studies comparisons.

The sol/gel transition temperature and time was assessed in triplicate by the measurement of time and temperature at which a magnetic bar stopped moving owing to gelation. For this task, a 10 mL sample was put into a transparent vial containing the magnetic bar at constant rotation speed of 400 rpm in a magnetic water bath from 4 to 37 ± 0.1 °C.

Scanning electron microscopy (FEI Quanta® FEG 650, Thermo Fisher Scientific-FEI, Hillsboro, CA, USA) was utilized to investigate the morphology of PLX/CS/HA-VM. Samples were processed using the critical point drying technique. PLX/CS/HA-VM was sputtered with carbon before observation.

The pH value of hydrogel was recorded using a digital pH meter GLP 22 (Crison Instruments, Alella, Spain) at room temperature. The measurements were conducted by direct immersion of the device electrode in the sample. Obtained data are expressed as the mean ± SD of three replicates.

2.3. Antioxidant Efficiency

The radical scavenging activity of blank PLX/CS/HA, PLX/CS/HA-V, PLC/CS/HA-M and PLX/CS/HA-VM was tested by measuring their capacity to scavenge the stable 1, 1-diphenyl-2-picrylhydrazyl (DPPH, Sigma-Aldrich Chemie, Steinheim, Germany). For this task, each hydrogel was prepared by taking 500 µL of the formulation and 1500 µL of the DPPH ethanolic solution. The reaction mixtures were shaken vigorously and then kept at 30 °C. Their absorbances were recorded in triplicate spectrophotometrically with the method of a slightly modified test of Brand-Williams [44] at 515 nm on a Spectronic Genesys 8 UV/Vis spectrophotometer (Fisher Scientific, Rochester, NJ, USA).

The percentage of radical scavenging activity (RSA%) was calculated according to the following equation:

$$RSA\% = \frac{A_0 - A_s}{A_0} \times 100 \qquad (1)$$

where A_0 is the absorbance of the control and A_s is the absorbance of the samples at 515 nm.

2.4. Antimicrobial Activity

The antimicrobial activity test was carried out by the Kirby-Bauer Disk Diffusion Susceptibility Test [45]. Gram negative bacteria such as *Acinetobacter baumanii* ATCC 19606, *A. baumanii* ABAU clinically isolated, *Escherichia coli* ATCC 25922, *Pseudomonas aeruginosa* ATCC 27823 and *P. aeruginosa* PAO-1 clinically isolated, as well as Gram positive bacteria such as *Staphylococcus aureus* ATCC 29213 and *Staphylococcus aureus* MARSA ATCC 43300) and fungi Candida albicans ATCC10231 were assayed. MacFarland standard suspensions (1.5×10^8 colony-forming units/mL) were used for each strain and then added on Mueller-Hinton agar plates. Then, sterile filter-paper discs (6 mm diameter) were placed on the surface and 25 µL of a sample was placed onto the discs. The agar plates were incubated at 37 °C for 48 h.

2.5. In Vivo Wound Healing Study

This study was previously approved by the animal research ethical committee 387/18 of the University of Barcelona according to Spanish law (Royal Decree 53/1 February 2013) based on the European directive 2010/63/UE.

The animals were anesthetized by isoflurane 0.5% at 5 L/min administration followed by an intradermal injection of Buprex® 0.05 mg/kg analgesic. The animals were supervised by a veterinarian throughout the study.

Firstly, the backs of the animals were shaved and cleaned with 70% ethanol. The rats were divided into groups of three individuals ($n = 3$). Skin burns were caused by a 1.0 cm^2 superficial contact area of cylindrical devices at 100 °C. The treatments were applied once daily for two weeks in the following way: Group I positive control, the animals in this group received no treatment; Group II, the animals were treated with 100 µL of PLX/CS/HA without antioxidant actives; Group III, the animals were treated with 100 µL of PLX/CS/HA-VM; Group IV, the animals were treated with the commercial reference silvederma®. The wound healing process (WH) was recorded by the measurement of the wound size and applying the following equation:

$$WH(\%) = (\text{initial wound size-final wound size})/(\text{initial wound size}) \times 100 \quad (2)$$

2.6. Histological Analysis

After the burns were induced, the study animals were euthanized by cervical dislocation. The skin of the burned areas was excised. The tissues were fixed for 24 h at 25 °C in formaldehyde and then washed with a phosphate buffered solution (PBS). The samples were then dehydrated by immersion in ascending grades of ethanol solutions and cleared with xylene. Once the samples were dehydrated, they were embedded in paraffin. To proceed with visualization, the samples were cut into 5 µm sections, stained with hematoxylin/eosin and mounted in a light microscope Olympus BX41 equipped with an Olympus XC50 camera (Olympus Co., Tokyo, Japan). A neutrophil quantification was carried out, which involved dividing samples into three parts and counting in three random foci of the dermis.

2.7. AFM Force Spectroscopy Experiments

For the AFM experiments, each skin sample was defrosted at room temperature and cut by dermatome (Model GA 630, Aesculap, Tuttlingen, Germany) into 400 µm thick pieces. After that, the 0.5×0.5 cm^2 pieces of rat skin were immediately glued onto a steel disc and rinsed gently with buffer and with deionized water to eliminate any surface contaminant. Finally, the sample surface was dried under a nitrogen stream. Each sample was mounted directly onto the AFM scanner located in a chamber with a controlled temperature and humidity to prevent water loss from the skin at 24 °C and 70%, respectively.

The AFM device consisted of an AFM Multimode IV controlled by Nanoscope V electronics (Bruker AXS Corporation; Santa Barbara, CA) equipped with a 15 µm piezoelectric scanner. Silicon AFM tips with a nominal spring constant of 42 nN nm^{-1} were used. The samples were studied in contact mode and in air, with a scan rate of 1.5 Hz and a scan angle of 0°.

For AFM Force Spectroscopy measurements, the spring constant of each cantilever used was determined using the thermal noise method. Hundreds of forces versus tip–sample distance curves were acquired in at least 10 different spots of each sample. The tip–sample approaching velocity was set for all force curves at 1000 nm s^{-1}. Applied forces F are given by $F = k_c \times \Delta$, where k_c is the spring constant of the cantilever and Δ stands for the cantilever deflection. The surface deformation is given as penetration (δ), evaluated as $\delta = z - \Delta$, where z represents the piezo-scanner displacement.

On the other hand, the rat skin elastic modulus (Young's modulus) was calculated using the Hertz model by converting force versus tip–sample distance curves into force versus indentation curves. The Hertz model is a good approximation to our system as it assumes indentation is negligible in comparison to the sample thickness, so that the substrate does not influence the calculations. Thus, experimental force versus δ data were adjusted to Equation (3) to obtain the Young's modulus [46].

$$F = E/(1 - \upsilon 2) \times \tan\alpha/\sqrt{2} \times \delta 2 \quad (3)$$

where E is the Young's modulus, α is the half angle of the AFM tip and υ is the so-called Poisson's ratio. In our experiments, α was 22.5° and υ was assumed to be 0.4 for a slightly compressive surface such as skin.

2.8. Statistical Analysis

The results were analyzed with one-way analysis of variance (ANOVA) to evaluate differences among mean values. Prism® software, v. 3.0 (GraphPad Software, Inc., San Diego, CA, USA) was used. A p-value < 0.05 was considered statistically significant.

3. Results

3.1. Characterization

The developed hydrogel showed a whitish hue and a homogeneous and fluid appearance, with a temperature-dependent sol-gel transition at 30 ± 0.2 °C after 1.7 ± 0.1 min. The hydrogel was a free-flowing sol at low temperature (measurements started from 18 °C) and turned into a non-flowing gel above 30 °C (Figure 1). The obtained pH of PLX/CS/HA-VM was 5.0 ± 0.1.

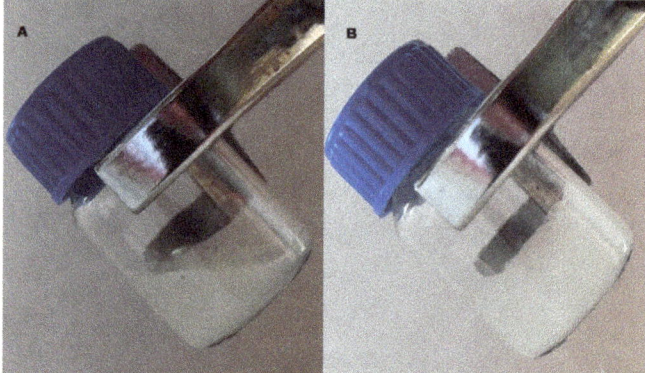

Figure 1. (**A**) PLX/CS/HA-VM at 18 °C; (**B**) PLX/CS/HA-VM at 32 °C.

The internal morphology of PLX/CS/HA-VM was observed by SEM. Figure 2 shows the internal porous three-dimension structure with approximately spherical and homogeneous micellar size.

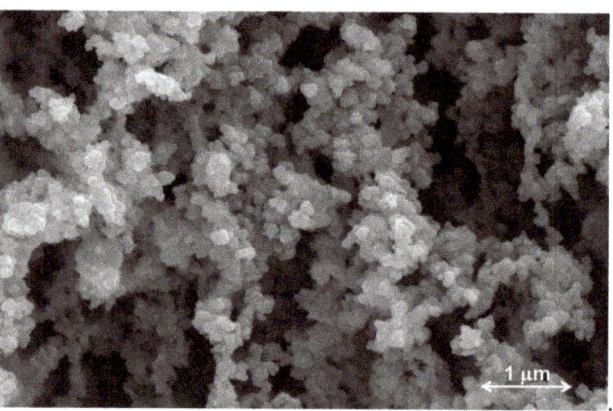

Figure 2. Scanning Electron Microscopy image obtained from PLX/CS/HA-VM, 30,000× magnification.

3.2. Antioxidant Activity

Figure 3 depicts the antioxidant efficacy results of the hydrogel loading vitamins, MLT and the antioxidant cocktail (vitamins A, D, E and MLT). As expected, blank hydrogel PLX/CS/HA showed no radical scavenging activity. Regarding MLT and vitamins, statistically significant differences were observed between both formulations, with RSA values ~18% and ~52%, respectively. However, the values of RSA for PLX/CS/HA-VM were significantly higher, in the vicinity of 70%.

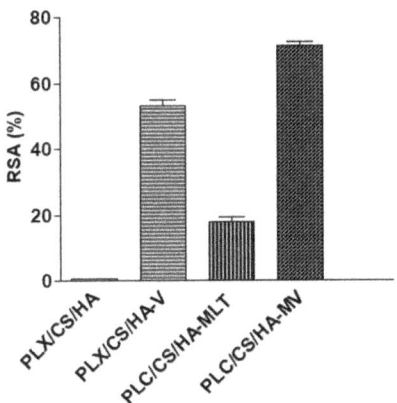

Figure 3. Antioxidant activity of hydrogels.

3.3. Microbiological Studies

Table 1 depicts the microbiological results of PLX/CS/HA-VM and the commercial reference against Gram positive, Gram negative and fungi strains. It is clear that PLX/CS/HA and PLX/CS/HA-VM produced significant inhibition of bacterial growth; they were roughly similar to the commercial reference, except in the case of E. coli ATCC 25922, for which both the blank hydrogel and the loaded hydrogel did not show antimicrobial action. Similar results were obtained in the case of growth inhibition assay.

Table 1. Inhibitory halos and growth reduction produced by PLX/CS/HA, PLX/CS/HA-VM and the reference formulation silvederma® against different pathogen microorganisms.

Microorganisms	Inhibition Halos (mm)			Growth Reduction		
	Reference	PLX/CS/HA	PLX/CS/HA-VM	Reference	PLX/CS/HA	PLX/CS/HA-VM
Acinetobacter baumanii ATCC 19606	7 *	8	8	+ *	+	+
Acinetobacter baumanii ABAU	15	10	9	+	+	+
Escherichia coli ATCC 25922	7	0	0	+	−	−
Pseudomonas aeruginosa ATCC 27823	7	10	7	+	+	+
Pseudomonas aeruginosa PAO-1	7	8	7	+	+	+
Staphylococcus aureus ATCC 29213	7	9	9	+	+	+
Staphylococcus aureus MARSA ATCC 43300	7	11	11	+	+	+
Candida albicans ATCC 10231	7	9	9	+	+	+

(*) Observed resistant colonies; (−) no growth inhibition; (+) growth inhibition.

3.4. Wound Healing Effect on Rat Skin

The wound healing efficacy induced by PLX/CS/HA-VM on rat skin burns is shown in Figure 4. Wounds treated with PLX/CS/HA-VM exhibited similar healing progress to those treated with the commercial reference silvederma®. After 14 days, a significant acceleration in wound healing was observed as compared with animals treated with the unloaded PLX/CS/HA hydrogel and the untreated group.

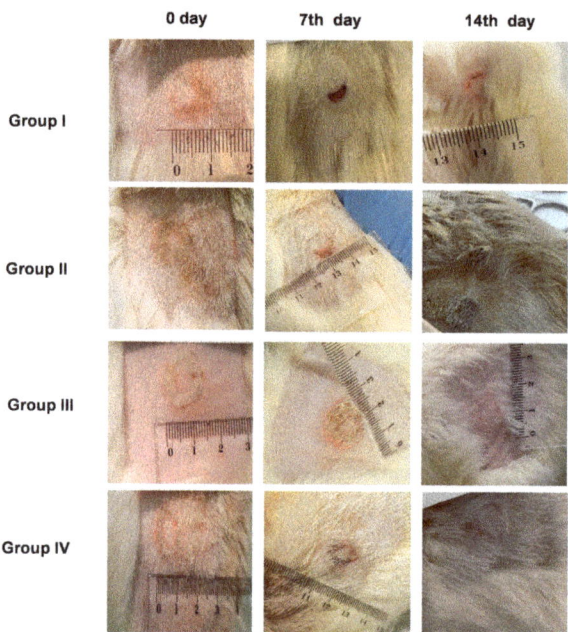

Figure 4. Wound healing evolution for 14 days in animals with no treatment (Group I), treated with PLX/CS/HA (Group II), treated with PLX/CS/HA-VM (Group III), and animals treated with the commercial reference silvederma® (Group IV).

On the other hand, wound closure was analyzed in each group as a percentage of the reduction in the wounded area after 14 days (Equation (2)), obtaining the following rates: 54.23% in the case of the untreated group, 63.52% in the case of animals treated with blank hydrogel, 96.12% for the group treated with PLX/CS/HA-VM, and 98.53% for the group treated with the commercial reference.

3.5. Histological Observation

Histological images of burn sites 14 days post-burning are shown in Figure 5. These observations were used to evaluate the healing potential of assayed formulations. In the case of untreated animals, an ulcer and the presence of inflammatory cells covered by a scab could be observed (Figure 5B). The tissue also showed increased epidermal thickness and a loss of epidermal appendices such as hair follicles. A similar pattern was observed in skin samples treated with blank hydrogel (Figure 5B), although the scabs were smaller. In specimens treated with the commercial reference silvederma® (Figure 5F), epidermis growth showing wound contraction could be observed. The groups treated with vitamin loaded hydrogel and MLT loaded hydrogel (Figure 5E,D, respectively) also showed a good recovery, similar to the commercial reference group. However, it seems that in conjunction they could ameliorate the regeneration of the epidermis and dermis, as it can be observed from the histological evaluation of samples treated with PLX/CS/HA-VM, in which both groups of antioxidant actives were included (Figure 5G). In this last case, skin showed less infiltration of inflammatory cells, smaller epidermal thickness and more epidermal appendices when compared to the commercial reference treatment.

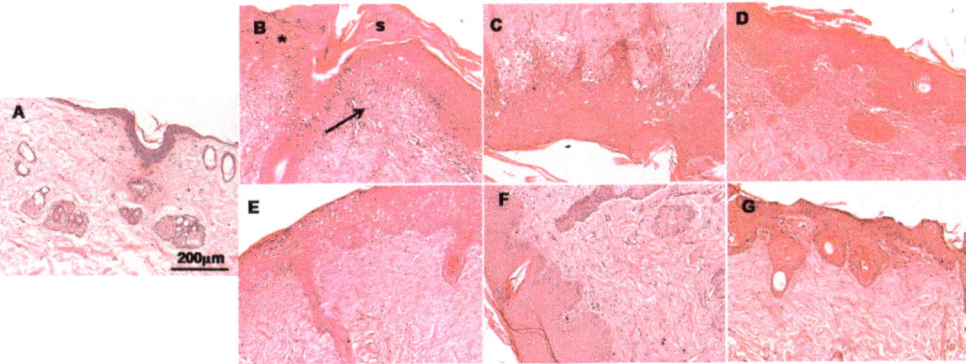

Figure 5. Histology of skin; (**A**) healthy skin; (**B**) burned skin without treatment; (**C**) skin treated with PLX/CS/HA; (**D**) skin treated with PLX/CS/HA-V; (**E**) skin treated with PLX/CS/HA-M; (**F**) skin treated with commercial reference; (**G**) skin treated with PLX/CS/HA-VM. Hematoxylin and eosin stains nuclei blue/black while keratin and cytoplasm are stained red. The asterisk indicates loss of stratum corneum and the arrow indicates infiltration of inflammatory cells, s = scar. Scale bar = 200 µm.

3.6. Atomic Force Microscopy

Figure 6 shows representative images of the health of rat skin under study. Figure 6A shows an optical image of clean regions without any detached scales or hair. Brighter zones were preferred over darker ones (intercellular gaps) to avoid any border effect. Figure 6A shows the three-dimensional (3D) topographic view of rat skin surface corresponding to one of the brighter areas displayed in Figure 6A. Some random structures ~500 nm wide with mean height values of 50–100 nm can be observed, but no keratin fibrils or organized structures were detected. As the scan size of this image is ~15 × 15 µm^2, the picture is equivalent to one fraction of the surface of a corneocyte. Furthermore, Figure 6A shows the corresponding deflection AFM image derived from Figure 6B. This image highlights the border of the scanned structures and reveals the roughness due to corneocyte disposition typical of healthy skin [47]. Furthermore, the friction AFM image of skin is shown in Figure 6D to assure the cleanliness of the evaluated sample, from which it can be observed that no changes in color are recorded. This is indicative that no lipids or other contaminants are present in the surface of the skin under study.

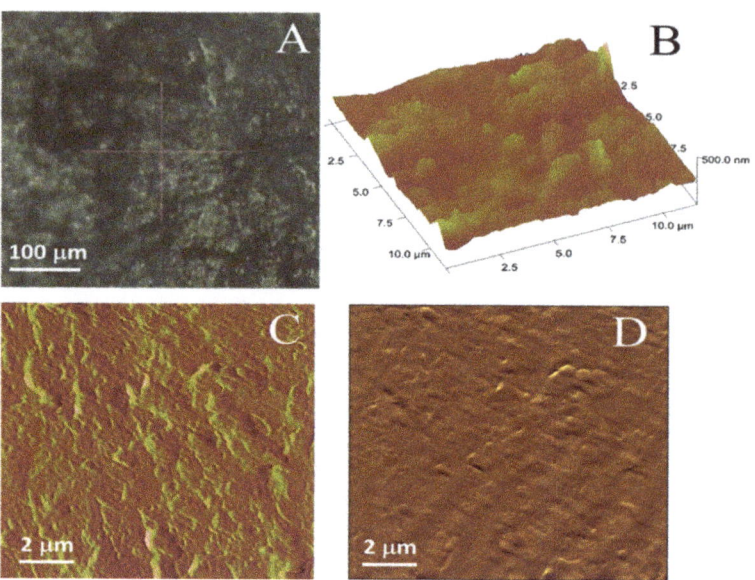

Figure 6. (**A**) Representative images for healthy rat skin as seen in the optical microscope; (**B**) 3D Atomic Force Microscopy (AFM) topographic view; (**C**) AFM deflection error image; (**D**) AFM friction image.

Young's Modulus from AFM Force Spectroscopy

Before obtaining force–distance curves to evaluate the Young's modulus, each sample was visualized to assure a 5 × 5 µm^2 homogeneous flat area, without contaminants or unattached flakes. Figure 7 shows histograms of the Young's modulus magnitude for healthy skin (Figure 7A) and burned skin without treatment (Figure 7B). It can clearly be seen that healthy skin presents a maximum (25%) at 104 ± 4 MPa, as expected, indicative of healthy rat skin presenting the highest Young's modulus value in the range of 0–200 MPa. It is also possible to observe a second peak at 550 MPa, but it is much less intense and diffuse, with frequency values around 5%. These Young's modulus values are quite high when compared with cells or tissues. In these, Young's modulus values are around 10–100 kPa [48]. However, the stratum corneum is more rigid than individual cells or tissues, and our values are in agreement with those reported by other similar studies with skin [49].

On the contrary, when the rat skin is damaged (Figure 7B), the maximum observed in the natural skin has almost vanished together with a shift towards higher values (190 MPa). The second peak in Figure 7B is also shifted toward higher Young's modulus values and spread in a wider range of values. Although it is difficult to attribute the peak, the mathematical fitting of the data to a normal distribution centers the peak at 1700 MPa.

The mechanism in which the stiffness of the damaged rat skin was modified after some treatments was also evaluated. Figure 8 shows histograms of the Young's modulus for blank hydrogel PLX/CS/HA (Figure 8A), PLX/CS/HA-V (Figure 8B) and PLX/CS/HA-M (Figure 8C). As expected, the treatment with PLX/CS/HA did not significantly modify the Young's modulus distribution when compared with burned skin (Figure 7B). Surprisingly, the PLX/CS/HA-V, although it has demonstrated some wound healing efficacy in previous studies [17], did not differ significantly from the untreated damaged skin (Figure 7B). Interestingly, the treatment with PLX/CS/HA-M (Figure 8C) partially recovers the main peak found in the normal skin (Figure 7A) but with less frequency, as there are still some regions with high Young's modulus values.

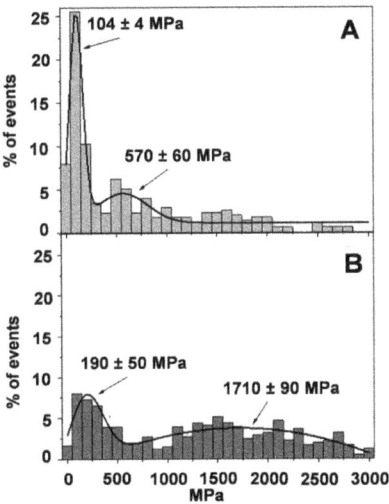

Figure 7. Young's moduli distribution obtained by means of AFM Force Spectroscopy; (**A**) healthy skin; (**B**) burned skin. Continuous line is the fitting of the experimental data to normal distributions.

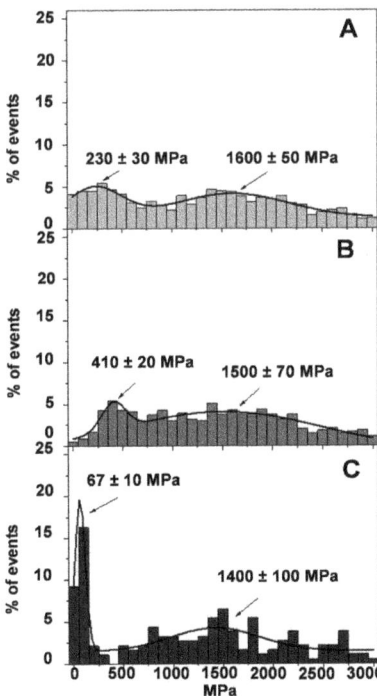

Figure 8. Young's moduli distribution obtained by means of AFM Force Spectroscopy; (**A**) burned skin treated with PLX/CS/HA; (**B**) burned skin treated with PLX/CS/HA-V; (**C**) burned skin treated with PLX/CS/HA-M. Continuous line is the fitting of the experimental data to normal distributions.

Figure 9A shows the effect of the commercial reference formulation silvederma® on the skin. The recovering of the main peak of the Young's modulus in the region 100−200 MPa can be observed, as in Figure 7A. Moreover, the second peak is also close to that observed in healthy skin at 570 MPa. The effect of PLX/CS/HA-VM, which is depicted in Figure 9B, is of great interest. The main peak observed in healthy skin is recovered, although with a lower frequency value (17%) and a little bit higher as it is centered in the region of 100–300 MPa. It is also possible to observe that the distribution of the Young's modulus at high values is decreased and a second peak seems to appear close to the 670 MPa. It is not far away from that observed in healthy skin or the skin treated with the commercial reference silvederma®. It is important to remember that PLX/CS/HA-V (Figure 8B) and PLX/CS/HA-M (Figure 8C) were not capable of recovering the elasticity profile of healthy skin, but the combination of both vitamins and MLT seems to be able to reach more than a significant recovering of the surface properties of natural rat skin.

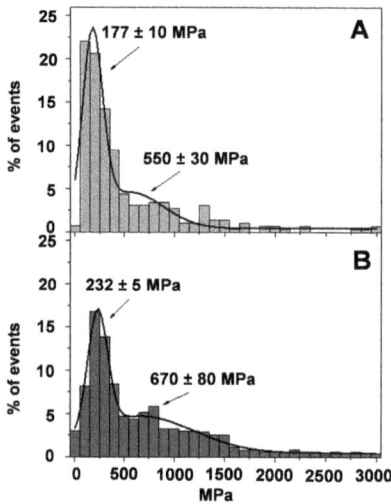

Figure 9. Young's moduli distribution obtained by means of AFM Force Spectroscopy; (**A**) burned skin treated with commercial reference; (**B**) burned skin treated with PLX/CS/HA-VM. Continuous line is the fitting of the experimental data to normal distributions.

4. Discussion

In previous studies [17,36], we evaluated separately the effect of vitamins A, D, E and MLT formulated in hydrogel of PLX, CS and HA aimed for skin wound healing. They evidenced great healing properties on induced skin burns, while being biocompatible with healthy skin. In the present study, we go a step further and investigate the effect of the combination of both vitamins A, D, E and MLT by using the previously developed hydrogel. Hydrogels are 3-D cross-linked polymeric networks with the ability to uptake a high amount of water or biological fluid [50]. In this context, the physicochemical properties of this formulation revealed a temperature dependant behavior due to PLX. Below gelation temperature, the formulation was in sol state (Figure 1A). PLX is a non-ionic tri-block copolymer of hydrophilic polyethylene oxide and hydrophobic polypropylene oxide. At a low temperature, the polymer molecules are encircled by a hydration layer in aqueous solution. However, as the temperature rises, the rupture of hydrogen bonds between solvent and hydrophilic chains takes place, and therefore hydrophobic interaction between polyoxypropylene units increases, leading to gel formation (Figure 1B) [51]. This circumstance is particularly interesting for administration purposes because it could be applied as sol state in the affected skin area and become a gel at physiological temperature, avoiding rubbing, pain or contamination and making the adherence to the wound easier.

On the other hand, the pH of topical formulations plays an important role with significant implications [52]. The pH of PLX/CS/HA-VM was 5.0 ± 0.1. This value can be considered an optimal value considering that the pH of healthy skin is around 4.7 [53]. This acidic medium provides a defense barrier against bacterial expansion and improves fibroblast growth [54]. Finally, the internal structure of PLX/CS/HA-VM, as shown in Figure 2, provides an interconnected channel structure, which was probably caused by the cubic self-assembly of micellar PLX [38]. It can serve as a reservoir for exudates. Rough surfaces may be caused by the action of CS [55].

The use of antioxidant actives such as vitamins A, D, E and MLT was aimed to counter the consequences of oxidative stress at the wound's surface. The combination of MLT and vitamins suggests a synergistic effect. The antioxidant activity of PLX/CS/HA-VM in terms of RSA was around 70% (Figure 3). This antioxidant activity has been demonstrated to provide a clear beneficial effect on the wound healing process by regulating the overproduction of ROS [56]. In the same context, the antibacterial activity of PLX/CS/HA-VM is also an important factor for skin wound healing, because bacterial infections can increase exudates formation and delay the wound healing process. Furthermore, the reduction in pathogens at the wound area also avoids the inflammatory response [57]. As depicted in Table 1, PLX/CS/HA-VM possessed antibacterial action similar to the commercial reference silvederma® containing silver sulfadiazine, except for *E. coli*. This action might be due to ingredients such as PLX and CS, whose antimicrobial properties have been previously described [27,58], and active ingredients such as MLT, which possesses intracellular chelator action. Despite these results, this antimicrobial action cannot be considered as an antibiotic agent, but it demonstrated huge potential to efficiently prevent the wound from bacterial infection and, thus, might provide a synergistic effect, acting like a disinfectant to the wound healing action of vitamins.

The wound healing performance of PLX/CS/HA-VM was further investigated by in vivo tests (Figure 4). As the wound healing process involves extensive oxidative stress to the system, an antioxidant cocktail was applied for promoting skin wound healing. There were no statistically significant differences in wound healing efficacy in terms of percentage of wound reduction after 14 days between PLX/CS/HA-VM and silvederma®. The latter is a topical antibiotic used in partial thickness and full thickness burns to prevent infection. This event revealed the wound healing potential of PLX/CS/HA-VM objectively. For a deeper analysis, histological studies were accomplished. It was observed that skin treated with PLX/CS/HA-VM showed less infiltration of inflammatory cells, smaller epidermal thickness and more epidermal appendices when compared to the commercial reference treatment (Figure 5). These results were in line with other studies reporting the wound healing potential of vitamins and MLT. However, apart from their antioxidant properties, the mechanisms of actions through which assayed vitamins exert the healing action are confusing and controversial [59–61]. On the other hand, antiapoptotic and p53-inhibitory processes seem to be involved in the healing mechanism of MLT [62].

In the present study, the possibility of using AFM as a complementary technique to evaluate the skin properties after induced burns was also investigated. It was found that damaged skin showed higher Young's modulus values, and this is indicative of stiffer regions. As expected, after burn heat exposition, the tissue could present an accumulation of liquids that rigidify the tissue, and although the liquid is progressively drained, it could remain in the wound for weeks. It is also possible that there was an increase in the epidermal thickness due to the wound caused by the burn, as it was observed in the histological frames. When PLX/CS/HA-V was applied on burned skin, no significant changes were observed. The distribution of Young's modulus values was quite similar to that of untreated skin or the skin treated with PLX/CS/HA. It was surprising that in previous investigations [17] the hydrogel containing vitamins A, D and E showed good results on healing burn wounds. It is worth mentioning here that AFM is a surface microscope and it can infer information about the surface of the skin or how the region beneath this surface can modify its properties. This means that previous results are not contradictory with these found now. In fact, the tissue heals from the bottom to the surface, so the surface is the last region to be restored. The vitamins used are soluble in organic solvents as evidenced by their log p values, which are 5.68, 7.50 and 12.2, for vitamin A, D and E, respectively [63]. Therefore, these vitamins are quite hydrophobic, and they could easily permeate through the stratum corneum to reach the epidermis where the healing of the tissue could start. If vitamins are not retained in the skin's surface, it is possible that the mechanical properties of burned skin would not have been restored, at least at the nanoscale.

Conversely, a different result was observed in the case of MLT. Previous studies showed the goodness of the formulation and the Young's modulus analysis also evidenced this effect. The partial recovering of the Young's modulus profile revealed that PLX/CS/HA-M was effective in the healing process of the wound (Figure 8C), or at least the surface of the skin and the surrounding area, as the skin treated with the PLX/CS/HA-M partially recovered the elastic properties of normal skin. MLT is a low water-soluble molecule, but its log p value is 1.18 [63]. Making a comparison between MLT and vitamins, it is possible that MLT molecules might remain in a higher concentration in the stratum corneum, promoting the healing of the wound. It is also presumed that MLT could permeate through the stratum corneum in a higher proportion; this can allow it to reach the epidermis layer.

To go deeply into the treatment of burned rat skin, the commercial reference formulation silvederma® was compared with the hydrogel loading antioxidant cocktail PLX/CS/HA-VM. The observed effect of PLX/CS/HA-VM was of great interest. In this case, the recovering of the Young's modulus profile indicates that the formulation is effective in healing the wound, or it at least shows comparable efficacy to skin treated with silvederma®. This correlates well with the histological results, where epidermal thickness was reduced, with less infiltration of inflammatory cells. The wound healing effect of PLX/CS/HA-VM could be due to the combination of the regeneration of the epidermis (vitamins and MLT) and the stratum corneum (MLT).

5. Conclusions

In this work, we demonstrated the significant wound healing effect of an antioxidant cocktail composed of vitamins A, D, E and MLT loaded in thermo sensitive hydrogel for the treatment of skin wounds. The formulation showed antibacterial, antioxidant action and enhanced the wound healing process in burned rat skin. In addition, in vivo and histological studies AFM Force Spectroscopy was employed for the analysis of the mechanical properties of rat skin. The combination of AFM with other common techniques such as histology or oxidative stress could improve understanding of the healing processes of the skin.

Author Contributions: A.C.C. and B.C. conceived and designed all the experiments, analyzed the data/results and wrote the paper; J.L.S. carried out experiments, analyzed the data/results, and wrote the paper; M.J.R.-L. realized the histological, analyzed the data/results; Ò.D. performed the skin evaluation by atomic force microscopy, analyzed the data/results; N.B.-d.F. carried out microbiological studies, analyzed the data/results; M.L.G.-R. conducted antioxidant studies, analyzed the data/results. All authors have read and agreed to the published version of the manuscript.

Funding: This research received no external funding.

Institutional Review Board Statement: Not applicable.

Informed Consent Statement: Not applicable.

Data Availability Statement: No new data were created or analyzed in this study. Data sharing is not applicable to this article.

Acknowledgments: The authors would like to thank AG Sanding and L Gómez from the animal facility (University of Barcelona) for his valuable help in animal studies.

Conflicts of Interest: The authors declare no conflict of interest.

References

1. Eyerich, S.; Eyerich, K.; Traidl-Hoffmann, C.; Biedermann, T. Cutaneous barriers and skin immunity: Differentiating a connected network. *Trends Immunol.* **2018**, *39*, 315–327. [CrossRef] [PubMed]
2. Rose, L.F.; Chan, R.K. The burn wound microenvironment. *Adv. Wound Care* **2016**, *5*, 106–118. [CrossRef] [PubMed]
3. Parihar, A.; Parihar, M.S.; Milner, S.; Bhat, S. Oxidative stress and anti-oxidative mobilization in burn injury. *Burns* **2008**, *34*, 6–17. [CrossRef] [PubMed]
4. Fitzmaurice, S.D.; Sivamani, R.K.; Isseroff, R.R. Antioxidant therapies for wound healing: A clinical guide to currently commercially available products. *Skin Pharmacol. Physiol.* **2011**, *24*, 113–126. [CrossRef] [PubMed]
5. Xu, Z.; Han, S.; Gu, Z.; Wu, J. Advances and Impact of Antioxidant Hydrogel in Chronic Wound Healing. *Adv. Healthc. Mater.* **2020**, *9*, 1901502. [CrossRef]
6. Zhang, S.; Hou, J.; Yuan, Q.; Xin, P.; Cheng, H.; Gu, Z.; Wu, J. Arginine derivatives assist dopamine-hyaluronic acid hybrid hydrogels to have enhanced antioxidant activity for wound healing. *Chem. Eng. J.* **2020**, *392*, 123775. [CrossRef]
7. Atiyeh, B.S.; Costagliola, M.; Hayek, S.N.; Dibo, S.A. Effect of silver on burn wound infection control and healing: Review of the literature. *Burns* **2007**, *33*, 139–148. [CrossRef]
8. Musalmah, M.; Nizrana, M.Y.; Fairuz, A.H.; NoorAini, A.H.; Azian, A.L.; Gapor, M.T.; Wan Ngah, W.Z. Comparative effects of palm vitamin E and alpha-tocopherol on healing and wound tissue antioxidant enzyme levels in diabetic rats. *Lipids* **2005**, *40*, 575–580. [CrossRef]
9. Di Lonardo, A.; De Rosa, M.; Graziano, A.; Pascone, C.; Lucattelli, E. Effectiveness of topical a-tocopherol acetate in burn infection treatment. *Ann. Burns Fire Disasters* **2019**, *32*, 282–288.
10. Wöbke, T.K.; Sorg, B.L.; Steinhilber, D. Vitamin D in inflammatory diseases. *Front. Physiol.* **2014**, *5*, 244. [CrossRef]
11. Scott, J.F.; Lu, K.Q. Vitamin D as a therapeutic option for sunburn: Clinical and biologic implications. *DNA Cell Biol.* **2017**, *36*, 879–882. [CrossRef] [PubMed]
12. Liu, P.T.; Stenger, S.; Li, H.; Wenzel, L.; Tan, B.H.; Krutzik, S.R.; Ochoa, M.T.; Schauber, J.; Wu, K.; Meinken, C.; et al. Toll-like receptor triggering of a vitamin D-mediated human antimicrobial response. *Science* **2006**, *311*, 1770–1773. [CrossRef] [PubMed]
13. Gronowska-Senger, A.; Burzykowska, K.; Przepiórka, M. Retinyl palmitate and oxidative stress reduction in rats. *Rocz. Panstw. Zakl. Hig.* **2010**, *61*, 21–25. [PubMed]
14. De Carvalho Melo-Cavalcante, A.A.; da Rocha Sousa, L.; Alencar, M.V.O.B.; de Oliveira Santos, J.V.; da Mata, A.M.O.; Paz, M.F.C.J.; de Carvalho, R.M.; Nunes, N.M.F.; Islam, M.T.; Mendes, A.N.; et al. Retinol palmitate and ascorbic acid: Role in oncological prevention and therapy. *Biomed. Pharmacother.* **2019**, *109*, 1394–1405. [CrossRef]
15. Malivindi, R.; Rago, V.; De Rose, D.; Gervasi, M.C.; Cione, E.; Russo, G.; Santoro, M.; Aquila, S. Influence of all-trans retinoic acid on sperm metabolism and oxidative stress: Its involvement in the physiopathology of varicocele-associated male infertility. *J. Cell Physiol.* **2018**, *233*, 9526–9537. [CrossRef]
16. Hunt, T.K. Vitamin A and wound healing. *J. Am. Acad. Dermatol.* **1986**, *15*, 817–821. [CrossRef]
17. Soriano-Ruiz, J.L.; Calpena-Campmany, A.C.; Silva-Abreu, M.; Halbout-Bellowa, L.; Bozal-de Febrer, N.; Rodríguez-Lagunas, M.J.; Clares-Naveros, B. Design and evaluation of a multifunctional thermosensitive poloxamer-chitosan-hyaluronic acid gel for the treatment of skin burns. *Int. J. Biol. Macromol.* **2020**, *142*, 412–422. [CrossRef]
18. Sierra, A.F.; Ramirez, M.L.; Campmany, A.C.; Martinez, A.R.; Naveros, B.C. In vivo and in vitro evaluation of the use of a newly developed melatonin loaded emulsion combined with UV filters as a protective agent against skin irradiation. *J. Dermatol. Sci.* **2013**, *69*, 202–214. [CrossRef]
19. Sánchez, A.; Calpena, A.C.; Clares, B. Evaluating the oxidative stress in inflammation: Role of melatonin. *Int. J. Mol. Sci.* **2015**, *16*, 16981–17004. [CrossRef]
20. Reiter, R.J.; Tan, D.X.; Herman, T.S.; Thomas Jr, C.R. Melatonin as a radioprotective agent: A review. *Int. J. Radiat. Oncol. Biol. Phys.* **2004**, *3*, 639–653.
21. Tan, D.X.; Manchester, L.C.; Terron, M.P.; Flores, L.J.; Reiter, R.J. One molecule, many derivatives: A never-ending interaction of melatonin with reactive oxygen and nitrogen species. *J. Pineal Res.* **2007**, *42*, 28–42. [CrossRef] [PubMed]
22. Rodriguez, C.; Mayo, J.C.; Sainz, R.M.; Antolín, I.; Herrera, F.; Martín, V.; Reiter, R.J. Regulation of antioxidant enzymes: A significant role for melatonin. *J. Pineal Res.* **2004**, *36*, 1–9. [CrossRef] [PubMed]
23. Wiggins-Dohlvik, K.; Han, M.S.; Stagg, H.W.; Alluri, H.; Shaji, C.A.; Oakley, R.P.; Davis, M.L.; Tharakan, B. Melatonin inhibits thermal injury-induced hyperpermeability in microvascular endothelial cells. *J. Trauma Acute Care Surg.* **2014**, *77*, 899–905. [CrossRef] [PubMed]
24. Pugazhenthi, K.; Kapoor, M.; Clarkson, A.N.; Hall, I.; Appleton, I. Melatonin accelerates the process of wound repair in full-thickness incisional wounds. *J. Pineal Res.* **2008**, *44*, 387–396. [CrossRef] [PubMed]
25. Pieri, C.; Marra, M.; Moroni, F.; Recchioni, R.; Marcheselli, F. Melatonin: A peroxyl radical scavenger more effective than vitamin E. *Life Sci.* **1994**, *55*, PL271–PL276. [CrossRef]
26. Korkmaz, A.; Reiter, R.J.; Topal, T.; Manchester, L.C.; Oter, S.; Tan, D.X. Melatonin: An established antioxidant worthy of use in clinical trials. *Mol. Med.* **2009**, *15*, 43–50. [CrossRef]
27. Carrascal, L.; Nunez-Abades, P.; Ayala, A.; Cano, M. Role of Melatonin in the Inflammatory Process and its Therapeutic Potential. *Curr. Pharm. Des.* **2018**, *24*, 1563–1588. [CrossRef]

28. Wang, H.X.; Liu, F.; NG, T.B. Examination of pineal indoles and 6-methoxy-2-benzoxazolinone for antioxidant and antimicrobial effects. *Comp. Biochem. Physiol. C Toxicol Pharmacol.* **2001**, *130*, 379–388. [CrossRef]
29. Reynolds, F.D.; Dauchy, R.; Blask, D.; Dietz, P.A.; Lynch, D.; Zuckerman, R. The pineal gland hormone melatonin improves survival in a rat model of sepsis/shock induced by zymosan A. *Surgery* **2003**, *134*, 474–479. [CrossRef]
30. Konar, V.V.; Yilmaz, O.; Ozturk, A.I.; Kirbag, S.; Arslan, M. Antimicrobial and biological effects of bomphos and phomphos on bacterial and yeast cells. *BioOrg. Chem.* **2000**, *28*, 214–225. [CrossRef]
31. Bonilla, E.; Valero, N.; Chacin-Bonilla, L.; Medina-Leendertz, S. Melatonin and viral infections. *J. Pineal Res.* **2004**, *36*, 73–79. [CrossRef] [PubMed]
32. Tekbas, O.F.; Ogur, R.; Korkmaz, A.; Kilic, A.; Reiter, R.J. Melatonin as an antibiotic: New insights into the actions of this ubiquitous molecule. *J. Pineal Res.* **2008**, *44*, 222–226. [CrossRef] [PubMed]
33. Romić, M.D.; Klarić, M.Š.; Lovrić, J.; Pepić, I.; Cetina-Čižmek, B.; Filipović-Grčić, J.; Hafner, A. Melatonin-loaded chitosan/Pluronic® F127 microspheres as in situ forming hydrogel: An innovative antimicrobial wound dressing. *Eur. J. Pharm. Biopharm.* **2016**, *107*, 67–79. [CrossRef] [PubMed]
34. Li, S.; Zhao, Y. Preparation of Melatonin-Loaded Zein Nanoparticles using Supercritical CO2 Antisolvent and in vitro Release Evaluation. *Int. J. Food Eng.* **2017**, *13*, 20170239. [CrossRef]
35. Li, Y.; Zhao, X.; Zu, Y.; Wang, L.; Wu, W.; Deng, Y.; Chang, Z.; Yanjie, L. Melatonin-loaded silica coated with hydroxypropyl methylcellulose phthalate for enhanced oral bioavailability: Preparation, and in vitro-in vivo evaluation. *Eur. J. Pharm. Biopharm.* **2017**, *112*, 58–66. [CrossRef]
36. Soriano, J.L.; Calpena, A.C.; Rincón, M.; Pérez, N.; Halbaut, L.; Rodríguez-Lagunas, M.J.; Clares, B. Melatonin nanogel promotes skin healing response in burn wounds of rats. *Nanomedicine* **2020**, *15*, 2133–2147. [CrossRef]
37. Sosa, L.; Calpena, A.C.; Silva-Abreu, M.; Espinoza, L.C.; Rincón, M.; Bozal, N.; Domenech, O.; Rodríguez-Lagunas, M.J.; Clares, B. Thermoreversible gel-loaded amphotericin B for the treatment of dermal and vaginal candidiasis. *Pharmaceutics* **2019**, *11*, 312. [CrossRef]
38. Maeda, H.; Kobayashi, H.; Miyahara, T.; Hashimoto, Y.; Akiyoshi, K.; Kasugai, S. Effects of a polysaccharide nanogel-crosslinked membrane on wound healing. *J. Biomed. Mater. Res. Part. B Appl. Biomater.* **2017**, *105*, 544–550. [CrossRef]
39. Müller, D.J.; Dufrêne, Y.F. Atomic force microscopy: A nanoscopic window on the cell surface. *Trends Cell Biol.* **2011**, *21*, 461–469. [CrossRef]
40. Jorba, I.; Uriarte, J.J.; Campillo, N.; Farré, R.; Navajas, D. Probing Micromechanical Properties of the Extracellular Matrix of Soft Tissues by Atomic Force Microscopy. *J. Cell Physiol.* **2017**, *232*, 19–26. [CrossRef]
41. Alcaraz, J.; Otero, J.; Jorba, I.; Navajas, D. Bidirectional mechanobiology between cells and their local extracellular matrix probed by atomic force microscopy. *Semin. Cell Dev. Biol.* **2018**, *73*, 71–81. [CrossRef] [PubMed]
42. Boughton, O.R.; Ma, S.; Zhao, S.; Arnold, M.; Lewis, A.; Hansen, U.; Justin, P.; Cobb, J.P.; Giuliani, F.; Richard, L.A. Measuring bone stiffness using spherical indentation. *PLoS ONE* **2018**, *13*, e0200475. [CrossRef] [PubMed]
43. Minelli, E.; Sassun, T.E.; Papi, M.; Palmieri, V.; Palermo, F.; Perini, G.; Antonelli, M.; Gianno, F.; Maulucci, G.; Ciasca, G. Nanoscale mechanics of brain abscess: An atomic force microscopy study. *Micron* **2018**, *113*, 34–40. [CrossRef] [PubMed]
44. Brand-Williams, W.; Cuvelier, M.E.; Bertset, C. Use of a free radical method to evaluate antioxidant activity. *Lebensm Wiss Technol* **1995**, *28*, 25–30. [CrossRef]
45. Hudzicki, J. Kirby-Bauer Disk Diffusion Susceptibility Test Protocol. American Society for Microbiology, Protocol 3189, 2009. Available online: http://www.asmscience.org/docserver/fulltext/education/protocol/protocol.3189.pdf?expires=1546990230&id=id&accname=guest&checksum=3BBDDB248802E16CC627C66E989A30E7 (accessed on 25 October 2020).
46. Lin, D.C.; Dimitriadis, E.K.; Horkay, F. Robust strategies for automated AFM force curve analysis—I. Non-adhesive indentation of soft, inhomogeneous materials. *J. Biomech. Eng.* **2007**, *129*, 430–440. [CrossRef]
47. Fredonnet, J.; Gasc, G.; Serre, G.; Séverac, C.; Simon, M. Topographical and nano-mechanical characterization of native corneocytes using atomic force microscopy. *J. Dermatol. Sci.* **2014**, *75*, 63–65. [CrossRef]
48. Kuznetsova, T.G.; Starodubtseva, M.N.; Yegorenkov, N.I.; Chizhik, S.A.; Zhdanov, R.I. Atomic force microscopy probing of cell elasticity. *Micron* **2007**, *38*, 824–833. [CrossRef]
49. Gaikwad, R.M.; Vasilyev, S.I.; Datta, S.; Sokolov, I. Atomic force microscopy characterization of corneocytes: Effect of moisturizer on their topology, rigidity, and friction. *Ski Res. Technol.* **2010**, *16*, 275–282. [CrossRef]
50. Souto, E.B.; Ribeiro, A.F.; Ferreira, M.I.; Teixeira, M.C.; Shimojo, A.A.M.; Soriano, J.L.; Naveros, B.C.; Durazzo, A.; Lucarini, M.; Souto, S.B. New Nanotechnologies for the Treatment and Repair of Skin Burns Infections. *Int. J. Mol. Sci.* **2020**, *21*, 393. [CrossRef]
51. Brugues, A.P.; Naveros, B.C.; Calpena-Campmany, A.C.; Pastor, P.H.; Saladrigas, R.F.; Lizandra, C.R. Developing cutaneous applications of paromomycin entrapped in stimuli-sensitive block copolymer nanogel dispersions. *Nanomedicine* **2015**, *10*, 227–240. [CrossRef] [PubMed]
52. Soriano-Ruiz, J.L.; Suñer-Carbó, J.; Calpena-Campmany, A.C.; Bozal de Febrer, N.; Halbaut-Bellowa, L.; Boix-Montañés, A.; Souto, E.B.; Clares-Naveros, B. Clotrimazole multiple W/O/W emulsion as anticandidal agent: Characterization and evaluation on skin and mucosae. *Colloids Surf. B Biointerfaces* **2019**, *175*, 166–174. [CrossRef] [PubMed]
53. Lambers, H.; Piessens, S.; Bloem, A.; Pronk, H.; Finkel, P. Natural skin surface pH is on average below 5, which is beneficial for its resident flora. *Int. J. Cosmet. Sci.* **2006**, *28*, 359–370. [CrossRef] [PubMed]

54. Jones, E.M.; Cochrane, C.A.; Percival, S.L. The effect of pH on the extracellular matrix and biofilms. *Adv. Wound Care* **2015**, *4*, 431–439. [CrossRef]
55. Ur-Rehman, T.; Tavelin, S.; Gröbner, G. Chitosan in situ gelation for improved drug loading and retention in poloxamer 407 gels. *Int. J. Pharm.* **2011**, *409*, 19–29. [CrossRef]
56. Zhao, X.; Wu, H.; Guo, B.; Dong, R.; Qiu, Y.; Ma, P.X. Antibacterial anti-oxidant electroactive injectable hydrogel as self-healing wound dressing with hemostasis and adhesiveness for cutaneous wound healing. *Biomaterials* **2017**, *122*, 34–47. [CrossRef]
57. Sudheesh Kumar, P.; Lakshmanan, V.-K.; Anilkumar, T.; Ramya, C.; Reshmi, P.; Unnikrishnan, A.; Shantikumar, V.; Jayakumar, N.R. Flexible and microporous chitosan hydrogel/nano ZnO composite bandages for wound dressing: In vitro and in vivo evaluation. *ACS Appl. Mater. Interfaces* **2012**, *4*, 2618–2629. [CrossRef]
58. Rabea, E.I.; Badawy, M.E.; Stevens, C.V.; Smagghe, G.; Steurbaut, W. Chitosan as antimicrobial agent: Applications and mode of action. *Biomacromolecules* **2013**, *4*, 1457–1465. [CrossRef]
59. Abdelmalek, M.; Spencer, J. Retinoids and wound healing. *Dermatol. Surg.* **2006**, *32*, 1219–1230.
60. Leivo, T.; Kiistala, U.; Vesterinen, M.; Owaribe, K.; Burgeson, R.E.; Virtanen, I.; Oikarinen, A. Re-epithelialization rate and protein expression in the suctioninduced wound model: Comparison between intact blisters, open wounds and calcipotriol-pretreated open wounds. *Br. J. Dermatol.* **2000**, *142*, 991–1002. [CrossRef]
61. Thiele, J.J.; Ekanayake-Mudiyanselage, S. Vitamin E in human skin: Organ specific physiology and considerations for its use in dermatology. *Mol. Asp. Med.* **2007**, *28*, 646–667. [CrossRef] [PubMed]
62. Milan, A.S.; Campmany, A.C.; Naveros, B.C. Antioxidant nanoplatforms for dermal delivery: Melatonin. *Curr. Drug Metab.* **2017**, *18*, 437–453. [CrossRef] [PubMed]
63. National Center for Biotechnology Information. PubChem Compound Summary. 2020. Available online: https://pubchem.ncbi.nlm.nih.gov/ (accessed on 18 November 2020).

MDPI
St. Alban-Anlage 66
4052 Basel
Switzerland
Tel. +41 61 683 77 34
Fax +41 61 302 89 18
www.mdpi.com

Pharmaceutics Editorial Office
E-mail: pharmaceutics@mdpi.com
www.mdpi.com/journal/pharmaceutics

www.ingramcontent.com/pod-product-compliance
Lightning Source LLC
LaVergne TN
LVHW070605100526
838202LV00012B/564